Solution-Focused Brief Therapy with the LGBT Community

Solution-Focused Brief Therapy with the LGBT Community is a practical guide for mental health professionals who wish to increase their therapeutic skills and work more effectively with LGBT clients. This book shows how to help clients reach their goals in tangible, respectful ways by identifying and emphasizing the hope, resources, and strength already present within this population. Readers will increase their knowledge about the practical application of SFBT through case examples and transcripts, modified directly from the author's work with the LGBT community, and by learning more about the miracle question, exceptions, scaling, compliments, coping, homework, and more.

Rebekka Ouer, LCSW, is a psychotherapist in private practice in Dallas, Texas. She specializes in the use of solution-focused brief therapy with the LGBT community, and she frequently conducts training for students and professionals on that topic.

Solution-Focused Brief Therapy with the LGBT Community

Creating Futures through Hope and Resilience

Rebekka Ouer

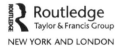

Routledge
Taylor & Francis Group

NEW YORK AND LONDON

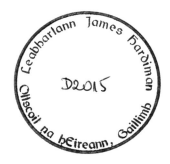

First published 2016
by Routledge
711 Third Avenue, New York, NY 10017

and by Routledge
2 Park Square, Milton Park, Abingdon, Oxon, OX14 4RN

Routledge is an imprint of the Taylor & Francis Group, an informa business

Library of Congress Cataloging in Publication Data
Ouer, Rebekka N.
  Solution-focused brief therapy with the LGBT community : creating futures through hope and resilience / by Rebekka N. Ouer.
    pages   cm
  Includes bibliographical references and index.
  1. Gays–Mental health.   2. Solution-focused therapy.
  3. Community mental health services.   I. Title.
  RC451.4.G39O94 2015
  616.89'14708664–dc   232015019872

ISBN: 978-1-138-81954-2 (hbk)
ISBN: 978-1-138-81957-3 (pbk)
ISBN: 978-1-315-74436-0 (ebk)

Typeset in Sabon
by Out of House Publishing

For MyShell; with every ounce of my love and appreciation

And for all of the sexual and gender minorities out there; this book was created with the sole aim of benefitting our community, and I dedicate it to all of you amazing souls who overcome the greatest of obstacles in search of the freedom to define yourselves for yourselves.

Contents

Foreword

Every once in a while I meet the therapists who offer elaborate praise and admiration for my mother, Insoo Kim Berg, and my thoughts often turn to "what would Insoo do if she were standing right here?"

Reading Rebekka Ouer's book offers a possible answer, and Insoo would praise Rebekka for taking on a tough but timely subject. She would also admire Rebekka for her absolute adherence to the SFT principles, most notably, respect for clients, which is evident in each chapter. While I don't know Rebekka personally, I can see she has such regard for her clients and that makes them lucky to have an engaged therapist.

As much as my mother would have rejected placing a name or a diagnosis to a client's problem (which she would have done strenuously!), she would have not regarded her clients by their sexual orientation or gender identity alone. As a lesbian, I am acutely aware that my sexuality is probably the least interesting thing about me; however, I am also aware that in the United States right now there is still conflict surrounding issues of sexual orientation and gender identity. Insoo believed in a person's defining their own self rather than being defined by others, just as Rebekka discusses in the opening chapters of this book.

I am struck by Rebekka's account of her calling for an appointment with a therapist who turned out to be "uncomfortable" seeing a lesbian client. Those of us in the LGBTQ community often have stories like this – a psychotherapist, family doctor, even a dentist who has "difficulty" dealing with difference. It reminds me of an experience of a female friend who worked in an all-male environment that was openly hostile to her due to her sexual orientation. She endured years of abuse, hostility, and discrimination and resorted to seeking counseling to deal with her enormous stress levels. The therapist she saw was well-regarded locally, however my friend discovered in the very first session that this therapist was just as discriminatory as her co-workers. That is why this book is vital to the conversation to end those awkward, disheartening encounters. More knowledge and awareness are the lights that shine on the dusty, old-fashioned ways of regarding someone who may be slightly different than you.

I hope this book is used by both professionals and the clients who are seeking a different outcome than what may have been the case with less knowledgeable therapists. Finally, Rebekka says that Insoo's work has changed her life, and I hope that Rebekka's work and this book will change the reader's life and as a result, the client's also.

Sarah K. Berg
Milwaukee, Wisconsin
May 2015

Acknowledgments

Michelle Lee – Because of your unwavering support, patience, guidance, and unconditional love, I was able to take leap after terrifying leap with my career. Thank you, I love you.

Elliott Connie – My career angel – You have been a Godsend to me since the day we met in 2003. Thank you for pushing me to do my very best in every aspect of my professional life.

The incomparable Rayya Ghul – Thank you for giving me (someone you had never even met!) a year's worth of the most helpful conversations I could have asked for. Your influence is all over these pages, and I hope I've made you proud.

My family – The Ouers, Desoukys, Fergusons, Mankins, Lees and Kings – Thank you for your support, and for cheering me through this journey. I love you guys the most!

Randi Hennigan and Jessica Demla – Thank you for listening and offering support and encouragement through this often-difficult journey.

Amy Phillips – Thank you for offering me the encouragement I need whenever I need it most and for always knowing exactly when that is. Love x 4.

Mason Tripp and Sheryl Fowler – You were the angels that God sent to help point my life towards this incredible path at a young age. Thank you.

My 'shipmates' –You all have a very special place in my heart, the confidence needed for this book grew its roots as I practiced alongside you guys.

This book was created with the help and support of a few other people, and with deep gratitude and appreciation, I thank them: Illayna Miller, Tim Cole, James Yeager, Lesley Worsham, Marc Coulter, Jose Jimenez, and Chris Iveson.

Introduction

The heart of human excellence often begins to beat when you discover a pursuit that absorbs you, frees you, challenges you, and gives you a sense of meaning, joy and passion.

(Terry Orlick, 2008)

My passion for solution-focused brief therapy

When I was little, and people would ask me the age-old question, "What do you want to be when you grow up?" I always answered in the same way, and the conversations looked a little like this:

Well-meaning adult: Hey Bekka, what do you want to be when you grow up?
Me: I don't know. I want to help people.
WMA: Oh, do you want to be a doctor/nurse/teacher? They help people.
Me: No.
WMA: So what *do* you want to be?
Me: I don't know, I just want to help people.
WMA: [shrugs and moves on].

Then, when I was 16, I was watching TV late one night, when everyone else in the house was asleep. There was an infomercial on, you know, one of those about saving the children in a third-world country, and I was watching it very closely. I remember being very interested in the show, and what people were doing to help the kids and families on it. They interviewed doctors, nurses, and teachers, and then they interviewed a woman who described her role with the kids and families, and my interest peaked. She sounded like she was working in a way that I would want to work with people. When her name came up on the screen, under it was the title "Social Worker." Right then and there, all alone in my den, I pointed at the TV and said aloud, "That's it! That's the name for what I'm supposed to be! Social Worker!" After that the conversations changed a little bit, and went something like this:

WMA: Hey Bekka, what do you want to be when you grow up?
Me: A social worker.
WMA: Oh. They don't make much money.
Me: Eh…I don't care, as long as I'm happy.
WMA: [SHRUGS AND MOVES ON].

Fast-forward to the summer of 2003: I was a year out of my Bachelor's program and taking a break from my Master's, working as a supervisor for an emergency youth shelter in Fort Worth, Texas, called the Bridge. My supervisors there sent me to a conference in San Antonio, held by an association known as the Texas Network of Youth Services. That year, the keynote speaker was a fellow social worker by the name of Insoo Kim Berg, a name that was new to me at that point in my young career, but one that would resonate with me throughout the rest of my professional life.

The first day of the conference, I remember sitting down early in the morning with a cup of coffee in a jam-packed auditorium, as I watched a petite black-and-gray-haired Asian woman put on a microphone up at the front. I didn't know it at the time, but the presentation that followed was going to make a huge impact on me.

I remember several things from that morning:

- Early on in her presentation, I realized that Insoo Kim Berg doggedly saw every single person she helped as an amazing and resourceful individual who was full of hope, skills, values, and unique talents.
- No diagnosis, nor anything anyone said about people or their circumstances, was capable of shifting this belief. In fact, it seemed that the more others tried to convince Insoo that a client was difficult or impossible to help, the more eager she became to begin work with that client.
- As I listened to her stories, and watched the session tapes she showed us, I realized that as she worked with her clients, she was more congruent in these beliefs than I ever knew a helper could be, even in the toughest of situations. Her questions held clear evidence of her beliefs in these kids and their families, and as they answered those assumption-filled questions, they seemed to be proving her assumptions right, over and over again.
- Sitting there and listening to Insoo, I remember feeling like she was a kindred spirit. And the most impactful piece of that day for me was hearing her say all of those things as a woman who had spent decades working successfully in this way with clients. She was living proof that one can have a successful career as a 'helper' and spend the entirety of it in complete congruence with these assumptions about people and the clients that they help.

That presentation served as all of the evidence that I would ever need that I could stay optimistic and hopeful for every client that I worked with for the rest of my career, and be successful at the same time. I now had solid proof that my own, seemingly naïve view of the clients that I worked with as amazing and capable people, could be preserved as I grew professionally. Insoo Kim Berg had unknowingly given me an invaluable gift in the form of permission to keep my hopeful and optimistic views, and discard the cynicism, bitterness, negativity, and judgment that already surrounded me as a young professional.

That day became a spark that slowly ignited a flame within me. A flame that helped me gain the momentum needed to introduce this book more than ten years later. It was the first of many glimpses I would have of incredible solution-focused workers like Heather Fiske, Tom Lee, Dr Sara Jordon, Dr Peter Lehmann, Yvonne Dolan, Chris Iveson, Harvey Ratner, Evan George, Guy Shannon, Rayya Ghul, Drs Arlene Gordon, Anne Rambo and Carol Messmore, just to name a few, who believe that you can trust in the best about people, and that you can work with them purely in that trust, without ever doubting or judging them, and be helpful at the same time.

About a year after attending that conference, I was working at a community organization also in Fort Worth. While there, I learned that some of my colleagues were studying Solution-Focused Brief Therapy in their various Master's programs. One day, after seeing me work with one of my clients, my good friend and co-worker, Elliott Connie, looked at me and said, "Bekka, you're *already* solution-focused, you just don't know it yet. You need to go back to school and study SFBT." So, I did just that. I went back to finish my Master's in Social Work at UT Arlington, where, in my practicum under Dr Peter Lehmann, I had my first opportunity to practice SFBT in a clinical setting.

An important point here, is that up until that time in my career, whenever colleagues or professors would ask me if I wanted to go into private practice, I always said "no." I hadn't ever pictured myself sitting in an office, opposite a couch, doing psychotherapy. I had always seen myself working at an agency as a supervisor, and maybe adjunct teaching at a local university. But that vision changed the day that I started my practicum.

Dr Lehmann is a proponent of SFBT, and as a result he trained his students in it, conducted supervision with it, and then challenged us all to use it in the sessions we had at the clinic. I knew this about Dr Lehmann going into that practicum, and as a result I was very eager to get started. I spent that year learning all about SFBT, the tenets, the assumptions, the kinds of questions and how and when to ask them, and then practicing it every single day, on a chair, sitting opposite a couch. I vividly remember walking out of my very first session at that clinic, having just spent an hour having a solution-focused conversation with a family. I walked out of the room and closed the door behind me (where the family was finishing up some end-of-session paperwork), and I fist-pumped the air as I thought, "I want to do *that* for the rest of my life."

As I continued seeing client after client at the clinic, I remember feeling like every single individual or family that I saw was proof of the assumptions that Insoo so clearly held for the people she worked with. The more clients who were able to answer these solution-focused questions about their hopes, strengths, skills, and resources, and the more they seemed to experience helpfulness through answering them, the more eager I became to continue learning and practicing this approach. I remember feeling as though (and often saying) SFBT fit me like a glove, and I began to feel as though I was born to work with people in this way. Those two semesters I spent at the clinic added up to one of the best years of my life. It taught me that sitting in an office, opposite a couch, doing psychotherapy, was *exactly* where I was supposed to be, and a few years later, in the spring of 2011, I began to work in private practice to do just that.

My passion for the LGBT community

In the fall of 2008 I was going through an incredibly tough break-up with someone I had previously been sure I would spend the rest of my life with. At that early point in our long and stressful separation process, I felt so confused and unsure of what I wanted to do that I called a therapist in my area to set up an appointment.

I spoke with a receptionist and explained that I wanted to come in for individual therapy with the hope of working out a conundrum I was experiencing in my relationship. The receptionist was very nice as she took my information, and scheduled an appointment for me early the following week. Before I hung up the phone, feeling a sense of relief that maybe I would finally be able to find some much-needed clarity, I thought that I should check about *one* more thing, just to be sure that I would be in good hands. I told the receptionist that, though I was planning on going into the appointment alone, I would be talking about my current relationship. I then clarified that the relationship was with another female. I asked if she thought that the therapist with whom I had just scheduled would be comfortable with that. I'll never forget the long silence that followed that question, and the subsequent answer, "No, he wouldn't be comfortable with that." I was stunned. Shaking a bit, I said, "OK, I guess you should go ahead and cancel that appointment." After the initial shock wore off, I felt a bit of relief that I thought to ask that question before walking into and paying for what had the potential to be an awkward and very unhelpful therapy session. But after that emotional experience I stopped seeking counseling for myself and decided that I should just try and work through that difficult time on my own.

I didn't want to have to ask that question every time I tried to schedule a new appointment, and I didn't want to risk dealing with the shock and disappointment that conversation made me feel.

As a direct result of that frustrating incident, three years later when I went into private practice I decided that my office would become a beacon for my LGBT (lesbian, gay, bisexual, and transgender) brothers and sisters. I wanted to do *everything* that I could to ensure that any individual, couple, or family in the Dallas-area LGBT community who was seeking therapy wouldn't even have to ask whether or not they would be welcomed in my office.

What I found in the coming months and years was that there are *a lot* of us in this world, and it is *incredibly* important to our community that we find help that is respectful and open to us. As I became busier, I realized that in any given week, 80–90 percent of the clients I saw were from within the LGBT community. I would often get feedback about how helpful it was that my office was so clearly safe and open to our community, and whenever someone was unsure about my office and it's openness to them, they would ask and immediately hear a reassuring and welcoming answer in return. I could often hear the relief in some of their voices after I answered their questions, further solidifying for me the importance of being a safe place for them to come and receive the help they were hoping for.

My biggest hope for this book is to help more therapists become both competent and comfortable working with the LGBT community, so that eventually folks within it can get the help they seek and deserve without ever having to question whether the counselor they are calling would be comfortable in their presence.

The intersection

At one corner of this intersection sits the LGBT community, and maybe more than any other group, our fight, our plea to the world around us, is to simply allow us to define ourselves for ourselves. All that we ask is for the right to define our bodies, our relationships, our genders, our attractions, and our families, with the same acceptance, rights, and privileges that are offered to our cisgender-heterosexual counterparts.

At the opposite corner sits SFBT, where the most important belief is that our clients are the experts in their lives. As such, in our sessions they get to, without exception, define their lives, hopes, preferred futures, preferred name, pronouns, bodies, relationships, genders, and everything else for themselves. It is because of this, as well as a few other guiding beliefs around SFBT, that it is my assertion that there is no more perfect fit between therapy style and clientele than SFBT and the LGBT community.

When I began working in private practice, specializing in work with LGBT individuals, couples, and families, I learned that there is something extraordinary and unique about SFBT when applied to this community. There are *specific* assumptions, principles, and solution-focused questions that I have with my LGBT clients that simply don't apply elsewhere. Coming-out stories became triumphant and heroic tales, filled with hope, strength, values, and resources. Relationships thriving despite not being legally recognized became hotbeds of resilience, coping, and togetherness in the face of adversity. Adults, unable to come out of the closet at home or at work, became people full of the most amazing coping skills you could imagine. And people who identify as transgender became the strongest, most courageous, open-minded, and self-aware individuals I'd ever had the privilege to meet. And in the conversations that we have in my office, those unique perspectives don't just become clear to me, they become clear to my clients as well.

As an openly gay clinician living in Texas, I am well aware that simply to exist as someone who identifies as LGB or T, you *must* have strengths, resources, skills, talents, and other attributes that have helped you move forward in a world that isn't always ready to accept your definition of yourself and your family. What I've learned through my practice as a solution-focused clinician, is that taking that knowledge and turning it into questions to point out and elicit the "how" of those successes, can be quite useful in uncovering and highlighting those strengths that can be called upon to achieve the hopes that our clients came into therapy with.

What's ahead

Chapter 1 introduces you to the LGBT community, and provides some unique cultural information and terminology that will be useful in a clinician's work with individuals, relationships, and families within it. Chapter 2 is an overview of SFBT and the tenets, principles, and assumptions at work within it, and within the intersection of SFBT with the LGBT community.

The format of the rest of the book, from Chapter 3 to Chapter 8, can be attributed, in large part, to Elliott Connie and his 2013 book *Solution Building in Couples Therapy*. In it, he breaks down a single session task-by-task and provides both insight into the task and a case study in the form of a session transcript that he sticks with throughout the book as a means of showing the reader what he does, how he does it, and the outcomes of his work. This approach to writing made so much sense to me that, with his permission, I took that model and applied it to this book as well.

Throughout this book you will see case examples in the form of stories, as well as one entire session transcript with a client in the LGBT community, broken down chapter-by-chapter. With the transcript, as well as the stories I will share about my work, I have, of course, changed the client's personal details and name, to protect their privacy. However, the rest of the transcript and stories remain true to the sessions as they happened. Throughout those chapters you will be taken task-by-task through an initial solution-focused session, with specific tips and examples for applying the approach uniquely to individuals, couples, and families within the LGBT community. Further, I will develop practical details on how to ask solution-focused questions and help the reader further understand the reasoning and timing behind those questions.

My ultimate aim for this book is to help current or future practitioners become more knowledgeable, confident, and excited about solution-focused brief therapy and its use with the amazing and unique LGBT community for which I am infinitely passionate.

1 The LGBT community

I think one of the marks of our profession is being very accepting of the other person, where they're at right now. That's been something that we try to instill in our students in our trainings. Golly, it's really hard.
(Insoo Kim Berg, cited in Yalom and Rubin, 2003)

The not-knowing stance

Solution-focused practitioners generally work from a stance of seeing clients as the sole experts of every aspect of their lives and situations, and thus we harbor a willingness to learn from them, especially those who are culturally different from us (Berg and Steiner, 2003). This core belief, one that has guided my work for years, left me wondering about the best way to approach this chapter. If you truly take on this stance of not knowing and allowing your clients to be the experts of their lives and their unique solutions, why would it be helpful to learn about the LGBT community in general? My opinion is that if you are able to be a blank slate, and stubbornly keep this not-knowing stance no matter what might come up in-session with your clients, this chapter may not be very useful to you. For some though, knowing what might come up, how clients might define themselves, their relationships, or their unique solutions, can help clinicians to stay more focused and disciplined with the solution-building process when those unique situations appear in their therapy room.

Further, sometimes, cultural norms and the solutions that are found to be useful with LGBT individuals, couples, and families can be *very* different from what those outside this community are accustomed to. Remaining a blank slate, then, might become problematic with this community if you hold a strong belief that homosexuality is a sinful lifestyle, or that being in a non-monogamous relationship is simply not as healthy as being monogamous with your partner. The clinician who holds these beliefs, or other beliefs that would challenge their ability to simply 'not know' with their LGBT clients, might find using SFBT difficult with this community. So as you read through this chapter, the definitions, and some of the unique differences found within this community, I challenge you to ask yourself if holding a not-knowing stance is truly possible for you in your work with this community. If the answer is "no," my hope would be that you would avoid working with this community until that changes. If the answer is "yes," than maybe this chapter will further your knowledge and allow that "yes" to be even more confident than it was before.

This chapter, then, will provide information about the ever-variant and evolving LGBT community, so that you can be more aware and competent with your knowledge of these clients, and how they might define themselves, their relationships, and their families.

If you are a clinician who works or lives within this community, this chapter might just be a bit of review for you; if you haven't yet worked or lived in this community, then I hope this chapter is useful as you learn what might come up in future sessions.

Who is the LGBT community?

I recognize that the term "LGBT" is limited in scope. It is, however, the briefest and most widely used and recognized term for gender and sexual minorities, which is specifically why I chose it over other options.

I want to clarify here that although the term "LGBT" is not all-inclusive, this book is about how to apply solution-focused brief therapy with *any* client who identifies as a gender or sexual minority.

So who is that exactly?

Sexual minorities

The term "sexual minorities" refers to individuals who are not heterosexual. This includes a wide range of individuals whose attractions vary greatly, most of whom are defined below.

Gender minorities

Gender minorities are individuals whose biological sex is different from their gender identity. This can include individuals who identify as transgender, demigender, agender, genderqueer, or something else. All of these are defined below.

The difference between gender and sexuality

I think the first lesson about gender and sexuality should always be that they are two completely separate things. The best way that I have ever heard this distinction explained is that sexuality is about who you go to bed with, while gender is about who you go to bed as. Somebody who identifies as a transgender male, for example, might identify as straight and only be attracted to women; they might identify as gay and only be attracted to men; or they might identify as bisexual, or any other sexuality as defined below. Until they tell you, there is simply no way to know a person's sexuality based solely on their gender expression.

Definitions

Throughout this book I will be using terms that you may not be familiar with, and in ways that might be different to how you have either used or heard those terms previously. I will list the terms I may use here, with definitions for your reference. This is in no way a comprehensive list of definitions within the LGBT community; it is simply a list of the current most commonly used terms, in my recent experience here in Dallas, Texas. The LGBT community is ever-changing and therefore the terminology is evolving on a regular basis, and it changes from day to day, city to city, state to state, and country to country. It is advisable for a clinician who works with this community to remember two important steps to keep up with current terminology:

1. Listen to your clients, and ask them how they identify or how they define their gender or sexuality. (There will be a lot more about how and when to do this in Chapter 2.)
2. Keep current on readings, especially with trusted resources on the web for up-to-date terms and definitions. Many universities have pages dedicated to LGBT terminology, what's respectful and what's out-of-date.

Sexuality Terms

Heterosexual: A person who is only sexually/romantically attracted to people of the opposite sex/gender.

Gay: An individual who is sexually/romantically attracted to those of the same sex/gender.

Lesbian: A woman who is sexually/romantically attracted only to other women.

Bisexual: A person who is sexually/romantically attracted to both men and women.

Pansexual: A person who is sexually/romantically attracted to people of any sex or gender identity.

Asexual: A person who lacks sexual or romantic attraction to any person regardless of sex or gender identity.

Thrupple/triad: A romantic relationship involving three consenting adults (typically male, but not exclusively).

Top: The partner in a relationship who is typically more dominant, and likely the one who is the penetrator, during sex.

Bottom: The partner in a relationship who is typically more submissive, and likely the one who receives penetration during sex.

Positive: Referring to HIV status, typically in gay or bisexual men, and meaning that they have been diagnosed with HIV.

Negative: Referring to HIV status, typically in gay or bisexual men, and meaning that they do not have HIV.

Open relationship: Referring to a kind of relationship in which each partner is free to be sexually intimate with individuals outside of the relationship.

Gender Terms

Gender: How a person self-identifies (i.e. male, female, genderqueer, etc.) regardless of biological sex.

Gender dysphoria: A diagnostic term referring to a feeling of discomfort within an individual as a result of a mismatch between their biological sex and their gender identity.

Cisgender: A person whose self-identity conforms with the gender that corresponds to their biological sex.

Transgender: A person whose biological sex is different from their self-identified gender.

Trans-man/trans-boy: A person who was identified female at birth but who now identifies as male.

Trans-woman/trans-girl: A person who was identified male at birth but who now identifies as female.

Genderqueer: A person whose gender is somewhere between male and female, and who may identify as male one day and female the next, or somewhere in the middle.

HRT – hormone replacement therapy: A form of therapy where an individual who identifies as transgender receives hormones of the gender in which they identify. A trans-male would receive testosterone and a trans-female would receive estrogen.

GAS – gender affirmation surgery: A surgical procedure wherein an individual who identifies as transgender, genderqueer, or another form of gender minority, modifies their body to conform with their gender identity and alleviate gender dysphoria.

Bottom surgery: Surgery in the genital area designed to create a body in line with a trans-person's gender identity.

Top surgery: Surgery for the construction of a male-type chest for trans-males, or for breast augmentation for trans-females.

Binding: When a trans-male wears a binder on his breasts to have a more masculine or flat-appearing chest.

Puberty suppression: The medical process of suppressing puberty for gender minority teenagers to ease gender dysphoria before they fully transition.

Important considerations for sexual minorities in therapy

Males and sexual freedom

One of the lessons I learned about working with the gay male community is that it is typically more sexually open than other communities. In one study of 566 gay male couples in San Francisco, 47 percent of those couples had an agreed-upon open relationship (Hoff, Beougher, Chakravarty, Darbes, and Neilands, 2010), while another study reported about 43 percent of gay male couples have openly had sex outside the relationship, (Solomon, Rothblum, and Balsam, 2005). So the lesson here is that open relationships are a part of working with gay male couples, and they have found numerous ways to make it work.

Women and sexual fluidity

Author Lisa Diamond (2008) addresses the phenomenon of sexual fluidity in women, and believes that for some females, sexuality is not rigidly heterosexual or homosexual, but fluidly changing throughout their lives. So what does that have to do with LGBT clients? Well, when you see a woman, in any kind of situation, it's important to know that her relationship doesn't define her sexuality, and further, that her sexuality today does not necessarily define her sexuality yesterday, or tomorrow. For example, in your work with this community you will likely speak with many women in lesbian relationships who do not identify as lesbians.

Important considerations for gender minorities in therapy

Preferred name and pronouns

Two of the most important things to consider with gender minorities in therapy are preferred pronouns and preferred name – which is frequently not their legal name, or the name that family members might call them. I'll offer some specific tips for obtaining this information in Chapter 2, but for now I'll reiterate how incredibly important it is to seek this information out, and always use clients' preferred names and pronouns.

Know why they are seeking your services

Adult individuals who identify as transgender and are seeking some form of medical or legal transition, often call counselors looking simply for a letter of support for the purpose of medical or legal transition rather than psychotherapy. There are many therapists who will only do a letter assessment as a part of psychotherapy. However, I do not believe this to be necessary, or particularly helpful to those of my adult clients who identify as transgender and who often don't want or don't need therapy at all.

So, whenever I get a call or email from an adult client who self-identifies as transgender, I always give them two options. The first is for therapy, and the rest of this book will be spent outlining what that means and how to go about it in a solution-focused way. The second option is a letter assessment, and the outline for that is a bit simpler.

Letter assessment for trans- and gender-fluid clients

A letter assessment is a series of appointments – sometimes as few as one, sometimes as many as three or more – where the clinician spends some time getting to know the client and asking them very specific questions about themselves, their identity, and their support system until the therapist feels comfortable enough to write a letter of support for the client's desired transition.

Sometimes the letter is in support of HRT or GAF, or it might be for a legal name and/or gender marker change. The questions in this type of appointment are typically centered around how long the client has identified as transgender, what extent of social transition they have reached, who in their life knows about this transition and fully supports it, whether they know of the permanent changes that will occur as a result of the transition, and an examination of the strengths and resources that will help them as they adjust physically, emotionally, mentally, and socially to this transition.

I have a form that I go over with clients where I fill in the information as they give it to me. My aim is to get as much information as I can, until I feel completely comfortable that the letter they are asking me to write is true. As soon as I feel that I can honestly write a letter of support for this client's HRT, GAF, legal name change, and/or gender marker change, I write the letter, sign it, and give them a copy.

Now, the most important piece of this is for a clinician to understand that a letter assessment is *very* different from psychotherapy. It is quite literally getting to know your client until you feel comfortable that you can write a letter of support for their desired transition (or, in the rare case that you are simply not comfortable writing a letter, communicating that with them and educating them about how they can move forward in some other way). It is *not* a therapeutic conversation wherein you are helping them move forward in some emotional or relational way. So, if you are doing an assessment, it is imperative that both you and your client know the difference, so that your client is fully aware of their options, and thus willingly participating in the session as it is defined.

Trans- and gender-fluid children and teens

More and more, children and teenagers are coming out to their parents as transgender or some other form of gender-fluid. When a family calls a therapist with this being the case, a letter assessment is not typically an option on the table. Medical providers who offer transition options to children and teenagers, such as puberty suppressants and eventually hormones, typically require that the kid be seen by a therapist for at least six months before medically transitioning, and then throughout the course of transition, until the teen turns 18. A letter is certainly a part of what a therapist can offer the family, but in this case, and at this point (unless and until the guidelines change), only as a part of on-going psychotherapy. Many times parents are thrilled with the requirement to wait and talk this out a bit with a professional, but sometimes the kids aren't quite as pleased. I'll talk more specifically about this type of situation as it relates to SFBT in another chapter. But I will say that as the numbers of these kids coming out has increased, and thus their presence in my office has increased, I have begun to offer group therapy, once a month or so, rather than just individual therapy, as a choice for them and their parents. Usually kids who have little or no interest in one-on-one discussions with a therapist for six long months are more than happy to meet in a group setting so they can talk with other kids like themselves and get a sense of camaraderie in the form of face-to-face interactions.

The LGBT community and resilience

Society's views on the LGBT community have certainly come a long way, and recently things have been changing quite rapidly. However, there are still very real struggles faced by this community. According to a 2013 report by the Pew Research Center, for example:

> a new nationally representative survey of 1,197 LGBT adults offers testimony to the many ways they feel they have been stigmatized by society. About four-in-ten (39%) say that at some point in their lives they were rejected by a family member or close friend because of their sexual orientation or gender identity; 30% say they have been physically attacked or threatened; 29% say they have been made to feel unwelcome in a place of worship; and 21% say they have been treated unfairly by an employer. About six-in-ten (58%) say they've been the target of slurs or jokes.
>
> (Taylor, 2013, p. 1)

I don't imagine much surprise when one reads these statistics, but what's significant here is the forced resiliency those numbers imply. When you work with the LGBT community, you will frequently hear of hardships resulting merely from identifying in this way. A natural part of the stories of these individuals is overcoming hurdles throughout their lives. Throughout the rest of this book I expand greatly on how a clinician using SFBT can use these stories to help their clients to identify and name the resiliencies, resources, values, and strengths they have successfully used to either avoid or overcome these obstacles so that they can continue moving forward, toward their preferred future.

A word about conversion therapy

Conversion therapy, or therapy involving a client within the LGBT community wherein the therapist sees their job as helping that person to become a cisgender-heterosexual, is simply *not* therapy. It should, in my opinion, be punishable anywhere it is practiced by taking the 'therapist's' license away and banning them from the ability to practice licensed therapy. As one author points out:

> In 2009, the APA issued a report concluding that the reported risks of the practices include: depression, guilt, helplessness, hopelessness, shame, social withdrawal, suicidality, substance abuse, stress, disappointment, self-blame, decreased self-esteem and authenticity to others, increased self-hatred, hostility and blame toward parents, feelings of anger and betrayal, loss of friends and potential romantic partners, problems in sexual and emotional intimacy, sexual dysfunction, high-risk sexual behaviors, a feeling of being dehumanized and untrue to self, a loss of faith, and a sense of having wasted time and resources.
>
> (National Center for Lesbian Rights, 2015)

Because of these incredibly negative effects, I believe that the licensing boards of all mental health professions should ban conversion therapy from ethical practices. Conversion therapy has been shown time and time again to be harmful, and in the helping professions our most important rule is to first do no harm. Deaths by many LGBT individuals, and especially youths who commit suicide, might be avoided by well-educated therapists helping individuals and their parents to understand what is truly happening and that LGBT identities cannot and should not be changed. I believe that when that doesn't happen, and a client attempts or commits suicide as a result, the blame, at least partially, lies with the therapist who was hired to help but instead tried to change that client and enforce the idea to them, their parents, and other loved ones, that identifying as LGB or T is a mental illness that can be cured through therapy and prayer rather than a legitimate state of being that can be adjusted to healthily through familial and social acceptance, and, for some, transition.

My hope is that the licensing boards of mental health professionals do more than just take a firm stance on this harmful practice. I hope that they outright ban it, and take the licenses away from any therapist who utilizes any form of conversion or reparative therapy.

Conclusion

So, what does all of this tell you about how to integrate this knowledge into becoming a solution-focused clinician skilled at working with the LGBT community? Well, the rest of this book, and in particular Chapter 2, will spell this out more clearly. If I've done what I set out to at the beginning of this chapter, you will by now know that simply allowing every single client that you see to define themselves for themselves, in every aspect of their lives and identities, without making any assumptions, is the most important piece of working with the LGBT community. And hopefully knowing some of the terms that might come up in your session with this community will help you to stay focused on the process of therapy when those things come up in session.

However, I warn you again that this is a community that is ever-changing and ever-variant, so one cannot simply know what there is to know today and expect that knowledge to hold true tomorrow. Listen to your clients, and to this community at large, when they tell you who they are – and don't be surprised when that definition changes or evolves from one client to the next, or even from one day to the next.

2 SFBT and the LGBT community

Listen to the questions people ask and you get a fairly good idea of what
they believe, what they value, and what they hope to accomplish.
(S.L. Witkin, 1999)

I was having dinner with my father one night after work, and we were
talking about my counseling practice and the way that I do therapy. I told
him a little bit about solution-focused brief therapy, and then I told him
that the very first question I ask every single client I see is something along
the lines of, "What would you like to notice happening in the coming
hours, days, and weeks, as a result of our successful work together?" My
dad looked down at his plate for a second, then he looked me in the eye
and said, almost accusingly, "Rebekka, there's a pretty big assumption
in that question." I laughed as I admitted that he couldn't be more right.
I then shared with him that I work from a *lot* of assumptions in-session
with my clients, and that those assumptions are what set solution-focused
practitioners apart from those who utilize other approaches. Insoo Kim
Berg and Therese Steiner (2003) addressed these assumptions when they
wrote, "Like all models of treatment, our clinical practices flow from
these assumptions. These beliefs in people we work with guide us at every
turn, even when we face situations for which we have no answers" (p. 18).

The question I shared with my dad actually holds several assumptions
within it. The first is that my client is coming to see me with hope. Second,
that they will be able to recognize those hopes being achieved, as soon as
they begin to achieve them, and they may notice it within hours of our
work together. And the third assumption within that question, the one
my dad was referring to, is that our work together will be successful.

Though I will delve into these, and other assumptions, in great detail
later in this chapter, I want to address the belief that clients come to us
with hope. Steve de Shazer once wrote that "Interestingly, you cannot
have a problem without first having the idea that a solution is possible"
(Zeig and Gilligan, 2013, p. 95). And if you think about it, you'll recognize that just the act of scheduling an appointment with a therapist, a

person whose job it is to help them, implies that a person has hope. And even when they are not the ones who have scheduled the appointment, their presence in a counseling office is just as evident of the presence of that hope within them. Therefore, just the simple act of sitting in my office lets me know that my clients are hopeful people. This assumption gives me permission to treat them as a person with hope rather than as a person with problems. This is an incredibly important distinction that becomes clear from the very first words that they hear me speak, words that I'll further delve into in Chapter 3.

You may realize by this point, as my dad did at dinner that night, that a solution-focused practitioner is operating with some pretty unique assumptions, both about people, and about what is helpful in therapy. As solution-focused therapists, we purposefully choose to spend a good deal of our time in-session tenaciously asking questions driven directly from these assumptions, over and over again. No matter who our client is or the problems that they have, we hold those assumptions close, and they carefully guide every single question we ask and every statement we make.

Solution-focused tenets and assumptions

So what are these assumptions that guide our every utterance? The following assumptions and tenets lay the groundwork for the practice of SFBT.

Tenets

If it isn't broken, don't' fix it

In the book *More Than Miracles*, the authors address this tenet by writing that "Nothing would seem more absurd than to intervene upon a situation that is already resolved" (de Shazer, Dolan, Korman, Trepper, McCollum, and Berg, 2007, pp. 1–2). And in the therapy room, if the client does not see something as a problem in their life, then neither does the SF therapist. There are many therapists who assert that just being an individual who identifies as transgender is reason enough to be in therapy, whether that individual wants, or thinks that they need therapy, or not. This tenet however, asserts that if a client doesn't believe they have issues related to their transgender identity, a solution-focused therapist would respect that. With this tenet as a guide, the therapist simply trusts the client's words and never assumes or attempts to address a situation that the client doesn't identify as problematic.

If it works, do more of it

Straightforward as it is, this tenet simply refers to things in the client's life that are working to help move them toward their preferred future.

This is another tenet that is incredibly important with regard to working with the LGBT community. Many times LGBT clients might have "out of the box" solutions that work really well for them. For example, I once saw a gay couple who solved one of their biggest relationship issues by opening up their sex life to other men, such that each partner had the freedom to date and be intimate with others outside their relationship. That couple developed an unorthodox solution for sure. However this tenet insists that the therapist trusts that their clients know what is best. That couple found what worked for them, and although it might not work for all couples, they were happier together as a result of continuing to do it. There are many therapists, of course, who would see that as an incredibly unhealthy way of living; however, with this unique couple it simply worked, and it worked very well. This tenet invites clients and therapists to simply notice what works, and to do more of it in order to move toward the preferred future that the client has come into therapy hoping to reach.

If it's not working, do something different

How many times have we all heard the saying that the definition of insanity is trying the same thing over and over again, and expecting different results? This tenet is very much in line with that way of thinking. Historically, therapists have been taught that if they offer an intervention to a client, and that intervention fails, the fault lies with the client's level of resistance, and therefore the client needs to fix their issue and try the intervention again (de Shazer et al., 2007). This tenet asserts, however, that if a client either tries a new intervention and it fails, or chooses not to try it at all, the therapist's job is to trust that the fault lies with the intervention and not with the client, and therefore the next step should be to simply do something different until the client finds what works.

Small steps lead to big changes

This tenet stems from a belief that I see evidence of every single day in my practice: that solutions snowball. In *More Than Miracles* (2007), the authors write that "It is assumed that once a small change has been made, it will lead to a series of further changes, which in turn lead to others, gradually resulting in a much larger systemic change without major disruption" (p. 2).

I remember working with a 16-year-old trans-boy who wanted more than anything to be more confident as a guy so that he could begin to socially transition at his new high school a few months later. Up until that point, he had still been going by his given name, Christen, and using female pronouns. So to start his transition, he asked his parents to call him Chris, and to begin using male pronouns in the home so that he could see how it affected his confidence. His parents and younger sisters were fully supportive of this desire, and within weeks they all noticed a huge turnaround with him at home. He was coming out of his room more and spending time with the family, even suggesting games for their game nights and actively participating in them. This spurred a desire to write a letter to some of his closer friends and family members, coming out to them and explaining what was going on. He got such great support from his loved ones that when school started, and with a little familial and faculty support, he was able to walk in as a teenaged boy, and with more confidence and happiness than he had ever felt, all starting with a small but incredibly meaningful shift at home.

The solution is not necessarily directly related to the problem

One of the most amazing things about solution-focused therapy is the truth behind this tenet. The reality of this tenet is an incredible reminder not to get too engaged in problem-talk, even when the client seems to be begging us to.

I remember meeting Michelle and Amy at the beginning of 2013. Michelle's adult son had recently begun living with them, and Amy was as frustrated with this living arrangement as she could possibly be. Amy made it clear during the first session that all of their misery was rooted in this issue, and unless Michelle's son left she was totally convinced they would have to separate. However, as we engaged in a detailed solution-building conversation about their preferred future, Michelle's son never once came up. Rather, the couple talked about spending time together and truly having fun again, doing things like going on hikes and to ball games, planning trips out of town together, and really prioritizing each other like they did when they began dating. They talked about increasing physical and verbal affection and intimacy, and socializing more with close friends. A few weeks later when they came back in for their second session, they were both incredibly pleased with the progress they had made. They were being thoughtful of each other and prioritizing their relationship, and things were better as a result.

During that session, Amy brought up Michelle's son, and I instinctively braced myself for the ensuing argument. But what happened next made me want to high-five them both right then and there. She said that throughout their time moving closer together in recent weeks, her mood had improved so much that she unexpectedly also got closer to Michelle's son. She said that she consciously made the decision to think of him as a part of her own family, and the result of that shift helped her to be there for him in such a way that she actually enjoyed having him around. She even began to notice the progress he was making towards independence, something she had previously not noticed at all. Further, she said that she was quite pleased with Michelle's very different responses to her son pushing some limits at home, which made her feel like Michelle was on her team, allowing them all to have calm and productive conversations about the situation, and work towards resolution while Michelle and Amy stayed firmly on the same page.

The point of this story, and with this tenet, is that solution-focused conversations lead to the revelation of a preferred future that might have nothing at all to do with "solving" the problem the client has identified. In fact, the conversation itself might never mention the problem at all. But when you move closer to your preferred future, solutions will snowball all over every aspect of your life. Therefore, engaging in solution-talk can be the quickest means of moving forward, and against all logic can actually solve problems that never once were brought up in that very conversation.

The language of solution-building is different than that of problem-solving

A natural follow-up to that last tenet reminds us that solution-building conversations are rooted in hope, desires, positivity, strengths, and resources. SFBT claims that clients can move toward their preferred future without traditional 'problem-solving' with their therapist. If you are engaging in a conversation aimed at problem-solving with a client, you are simply not, in that moment, doing solution-focused brief therapy. If, however, the language you and your client are using is future-focused, positive, rooted in desires, strengths, and exceptions to those problems, then chances are you are having a solution-building conversation.

The future is both created, and negotiable

One of the best examples of this tenet came from a client I worked with named Stefanie. She came in to see me for the first time after an incredibly conflict-filled few months with her partner, mother, and co-workers. She wanted to feel in control again, and be confident and calm as she addressed the tough situations that had arisen recently. She also wanted to live a life full of fun and time with loved ones, without arguments popping up at every turn. We promptly engaged in a future-focused conversation where she was feeling confident, social, happy, and calm. She went into *great* detail about how this version of herself, at her absolute best, would go about her day from the moment she woke up to the moment she went back to sleep that night. Stefanie described a version of herself that she truly wanted to be, where she woke up early, worked out in the morning, set healthy but firm limits with her colleagues and family members, explored the city sights with loved ones, and remained calm, patient, and self-confident during difficult conversations with her wife and mother. At the end of the detailed description we finished the session, and she went on her way.

The following week, Stefanie came back and I asked her what had been better since our last chat. She hesitated a moment before saying, "I know this is supposed to be about me, but I have to tell you something."

Slightly concerned, I said, "OK, go ahead." And what she said then almost brought me to tears. She said:

> When I came in last week I was more stressed than I have ever felt, but I left here thinking a lot about our conversation, and that miracle day you asked me about. I thought about it for the rest of that day and into the night, I think I even dreamed about it. And when I woke up the next day, I felt like that miracle had *actually* occurred. I wondered if somehow when you asked me that question, we actually spoke the miracle into existence. You just asked me what's been better? Everything! Everything has been better since that day.

Stefanie reminded me of how incredibly true this tenet is. No matter what you might have been yesterday, last week, last year, or for the last 20 years, you can turn on a dime, and create the future you desire.

Five basic SFBT assumptions

To go along with the groundwork of those tenets, I have outlined five basic solution-focused assumptions at work within every SFBT session:

1. Every client comes into therapy with hope for their lives and relationships

Having already explained a bit about this assumption, I'll just say here that in Chapter 3 you'll see exactly how this hope is sought, from the very first question a solution-focused clinician asks.

2. Clients come from a successful past, and thus are already armed with the strengths, skills, talents, resources, and values it will take to achieve their hopes

One of my favorite quotes came to me from Elliott Connie, who heard his friend and fellow SF-er, Chris Iveson, say: "If nobody is perfect, then nobody is perfectly imperfect either" (personal communication, 2012). Everybody has a unique set of strengths, skills, talents, resources, and values that have helped them along in their lives and relationships. And remembering that there are always exceptions to every problem – times when the problem is happening much less, or not at all – tells you that every client has a rich history of using those strengths successfully.

3. Describing their preferred future makes it more likely that a client will leave a therapy session and begin to create it

Looking back at the very last tenet above, and remembering that the future is both created and negotiable, this assumption addresses how we put that tenet into practice. In the first solution-focused session the therapist elicits a detailed description of the preferred future from their clients. This is very different than other models of therapy, where you might spend the first session completing a diagnostic assessment or delving into the past problems of clients. This assumption asserts that describing, in rich detail, what you want – rather than what you don't want – makes it more likely that you will then be able to leave and create what you have just described.

4. Clients are currently doing some things well in their life/relationship

When people are in highly emotional states they tend to use superlatives such as "I *always* feel depressed. I am *never* happy." Or with a couple, "We fight *all the time* now." However, a skilled clinician knows that these superlatives are simply not true. The difference between a solution-focused clinician and a problem-focused one lies in the very next question asked.

The belief rooted in this assumption begs the question, "When was the last time you felt even a little bit happier?" or "And when was the last time you had an opportunity to fight, but somehow you managed not to?" The reason for questions such as these is that the answer gives us clues as to how we might begin to move back to "A *little bit* happier," or "Getting along *a little bit* better." And in these clues lie the bits and pieces of the solutions our clients came to us hoping for in the first place. This assumption enables those sorts of questions, and reminds us that there are *always* times when clients are doing better, and within those times lies a direct path to creating the exact solutions they came to us seeking in the first place.

5. Clients can begin moving toward their preferred future immediately upon leaving a session

Remember the example of Stefanie, from before? Well rooted in her story is all the evidence one needs for the presence of this assumption. Clients sometimes begin to create the very future they've spent an hour describing in great detail to you, as soon as they leave your office. You'll see transcripts and stories throughout this book that will further outline the evidence of this assumption.

BRIEF and BRIEFER

An agency called BRIEF – headed by Chris Iveson, Evan George, and Harvey Ratner, and located in London, England – has become one of the most popular training facilities of SFBT in the world. People travel from all around the globe to attend their year-round workshops and trainings. Even though, as of yet, I haven't trained at BRIEF, as a result of first being trained in graduate school by the manual they created, as well as being quite close with and learning so much from Elliott Connie over the years (a student, co-trainer and close friend of the practitioners of BRIEF), much of the way that I do SFBT has been highly influenced by their contributions to the field. Throughout this book I consistently reference their writing, as well as Elliott's, as I explain what I do and how I do it. I've learned a lot from both their and Elliott's incredibly minimalistic approach to SFBT.

In their manual, entitled Briefer, *they describe SFBT as:*

- seeing a person as more than their problem;
- looking for resources rather than deficits;
- exploring possible and preferred futures;
- exploring what is already contributing to those futures;
- treating clients as experts in all aspects of their lives.

(George, Iveson, and Ratner, 2011, pp. 4–5)

SFBT and the LGBT community

When I conduct trainings on SFBT with the LGBT community, participants who are familiar with this approach sometimes ask how it is different when working with LGBT clients. The answer is simple; it is not *different* so much as it is specialized to the specific experiences and commonalities of the LGBT community. In his book about SFBT and multicultural clients, Johnny Kim (2013, p. 10) addresses how SFBT can be specialized with minority clients when he says, "There are opportunities to structure a session around solution-building conversations that build on a minority client's unique cultural strengths and experiences that can lead to solutions to the problem."

The difficulties faced by LGBT clients can be found in many books about working with them in therapy, and in many of these books you will find that the authors stress how important it is for clinicians to be aware of and address those problems so that they might bring them to light in-session. For example, one author writing about gay clients points out that, "tracking the manifestations of shame and internalized homophobia in your clients is imperative. As a gay affirmative therapist, you must know what to look for and how to help clients understand that it exists within them" (Kort, 2008, p. 31). However, I believe that it is *more* helpful, and therefore important, to be aware of and bring to light how those unique experiences and difficulties bring out the inherent strengths, values, resources, and resiliencies within the LGBT clients we serve.

Five solution-focused principles with LGBT clients

With the assumptions and tenets of SFBT as my base, I have outlined five important principles that highlight these beliefs as they pertain to solution-focused sessions with LGBT clients. These basic principles, along with a solution-focused perspective, guide my therapeutic conversations in every single session I have with LGBT individuals, couples, and families.

1. LGBT clients/relationships/families are valid and have as much chance of health and success as their cisgender-heterosexual counterparts

The LGBT couples and families that you work with deserve a therapist who believes in their ability to be fully healthy and successful. In his book, *Solution Building in Couples Therapy* (2013, p. 1), Elliott Connie writes, "SFT with couples requires the therapist to keep the discussion targeted squarely on solutions – and avoid any distractions related to the couple's problem story." In relation to the LGBT community in general, keeping the discussion targeted squarely on solutions requires an *unwavering belief* in the client's ability to reach their very best hopes. And therefore it is of the utmost importance as a clinician working with the LGBT community that you see these clients and their relationships as being as valid and healthy as their cisgender-heterosexual counterparts.

The unique situations you will come across with this community might be new to you – such as, say, a seemingly heterosexual couple where the male has just come out as bisexual to his wife, and although she might be struggling with this new reality their hope is to work through it and stay together as part of a committed monogamous relationship. That couple needs a therapist who believes in their ability to do just that. All of our clients deserve a therapist who believes fully in their true potential to have a healthy and successful life, and when you hold on to this principle you are likely to ask respectful questions that reflect this belief.

2. LGBT clients come into therapy with histories that are rich with evidence of resiliencies, strengths, values, skills, and resources

Every client that you see has some story to tell about their life, and in her book *Tales of Solutions: A Collection Of Hope-Inspiring Stories*, Insoo Kim Berg (2001, p. xiv, co-authored with Y. Dolan) writes,

> While many approaches to therapy involve helping clients to tell their stories, a distinguishing principle of the solution-focused approach is that the therapist empowers clients to retell their stories based upon their goals, rather than basing their goals upon their stories.

It is my belief that as a *direct* result of their minority status, an LGBT individual, couple, or family must be overcoming familial, personal, and/ or societal difficulties *somehow*, and with this principle as a guide we can both carefully listen for, *and* respectfully invite them to tell us, how they have done so.

Imagine for a moment that a 54-year-old walks into your office for her first appointment. This individual is a successful businessperson from a small town, with a wife and three teenagers at home. Imagine that although this client looks like a male to your eyes, and sounds like a male to your ears, they tell you that although they were identified male at birth, and have lived as such their entire life, they have known since the age of four that they were truly female. Imagine that this client goes on to say that she didn't know until recently that there was a name for such a situation – 'transgender' – or that there were things that she could do to move closer to her true self, such as taking hormones or having gender-affirmative surgeries. Think for a second about the strengths, skills, and talents it must have taken this woman to live through a life for 50-plus years feeling that way. Think about the values she must have clung to, to keep herself going, and to stay hopeful through the internal struggles she must have faced, day after day.

Then imagine that she tells you the secrets to exactly how she did that, how she got through it and found ways to be happier and more successful in her career, and with her beloved family, than she knew possible with these difficult feelings she struggled with. And think about how those strengths might come in handy as she begins to move toward the challenging and possibly terrifying – but incredibly reward-ing – road of transitioning medically, socially, and physically toward her true self.

Helping clients to effectively retell their stories with a focus on evi-dence of their resilience and strength in the face of adversity, allows them to begin moving toward their hopes – and to do so as a resource-ful, strong, and resilient person who has so clearly lived a life that is already filled with evidence that they have these strengths and abilities within them.

3. A client's LGBT status does not automatically correlate with the problems they are experiencing

This principle is a direct offshoot of the original SF tenet that "If it isn't broken, don't fix it." This principle asserts that you simply *cannot* assume that your client is experiencing negative effects of their sexual or gender minority status in congruence with working in a solution-focused way. As I pointed out earlier, many people believe that simply identifying as transgender is reason enough to need therapy, regardless of whether that individual wants or feels the need to go to a therapist. It is my assertion that this belief is simply wrong. I think it is akin to believing that all left-handed people should go to therapy because of the difficulties faced by their left-handedness; and further, when they do attend therapy, their left-handedness *must* be addressed in order for that individual to be fully and effectively helped, even if they don't believe their left-handedness to be problematic.

This principle reinforces the idea that as the expert in their lives, LGBT clients identify their hopes and their problems for themselves, without exception.

4. Until proven otherwise, family members of LGBT individuals have the ability and potential to evolve and change their thoughts and feelings after a loved one comes out

I'll never forget the session that I had with a man in his fifties who came to me with the hope of coming to terms with the possibility that his adult son was gay. This man was devout in the strictest of faiths, and everything about his religion told him that if his son was in fact gay, he would suffer both in life and in his afterlife. But this incredibly loving and dedicated father came to a therapist who he knew to specialize in the LGBT community, with the hope of responding out of love for his son, should he come out, and keeping their relationship strong and healthy through this potentially difficult process.

I realized that day that there is *always* potential for loved ones to come around and find ways to love and accept their LGBT kin, and even when every card is stacked against the odds, that love can prevail. I also realized that if this session had been with the son instead of his father, he might have tried to convince me that his father would and could *never* understand or accept that he was gay. This son might have limited his hope to that of either living in the closet and remaining close to his father, or coming out and never speaking to his father again.

A therapist who believes a client with this limited hope would miss a huge opportunity to ask a question that might make the biggest difference in the world. A therapist who knows that people have the ability to overcome any obstacle that stands in their way, however, might find herself asking this son about a future in which his father finally *does* come around, and how this son might notice the signals of that reality as it began to unfold.

In your work with the LGBT community you will, quite frequently, hear coming-out stories or even see loved ones in-session as they adjust to the news of their son, daughter, parent, or even spouse coming out. Oftentimes the loved ones of that LGBT individual may be struggling quite mightily as they grapple the new reality they are facing. It is important to remember that coming out is an often-difficult process, both for the individual who comes out, and for their family and loved ones. A therapist who remembers that even the most difficult hurdles can, in time, be overcome, will be more likely to ask respectful questions as though the absolute best of their client's hopes can be reached.

5. As experts in their lives, each LGBT client defines for themselves:

SEXUALITY

It is important not to assume anything about how your client identifies until they tell you. I once had a session with a young man who emailed me through my LGBT website – so my seemingly innocent and logical assumption was that he was somehow from within this community. When he came in to see me, it was in the back of my head the whole time that he was either gay or bisexual. His hope from our work together was to get over a recent break-up that was giving him an incredibly hard time. About ten minutes into our session, he hadn't yet specified the gender of the person he had broken up with, but still I found myself assuming it was a male – he had come to me via my LGBT website after all. But before I could embarrass myself by asking a question about his ex-boyfriend, he specified two things: his relationship had been with a girl, and although he was very much heterosexual he came to me, a therapist that he knew specialized in the LGBT community, because he had recently tried another therapist who ended up being a conservative religious man that he didn't click well with at all. He assumed that because I was a therapist who specialized in work with the LGBT community I must be pretty liberal and open-minded, and he thought we would have a *much* better chance of connecting and getting along, and thus having a more helpful conversation. I relearned the lesson on that day that under no circumstances should I ever assume that I know the sexuality of my client.

Another aspect of this point is that just because you see two women or two men in a couple's session, does not mean that they both identify as gay. Many times one partner may identify as bisexual, or even straight with an exception, and sometimes they don't label their sexuality at all. As the therapist asking questions you might accidentally stop-down an otherwise very helpful conversation by assuming you know how a client identifies and labeling them as such before they have had a chance to tell you.

GENDER AND GENDER EXPRESSION

With this community, gender and gender expression is sometimes as fluid as sexuality. It is extremely important to allow your clients to identify their own gender before you make any assumptions about it.

I was recently meeting with a new couple for the first time, and when I went into the lobby to greet them, I saw what looked very much like a heterosexual couple. I realized, after introductions were made, that they were in fact two women – one of whom just happened to be quite masculine. Later in the session, when I asked them if there was anything they'd like to know about me, the more masculine woman asked me if I had ever met another woman who looked like her. I told her that I had, both as an openly gay woman with many gender variant friends, and as a therapist who works closely with this community. I saw her relax immediately upon my answering her question – she took a deep breath and sat back on the sofa, as she told me that she had recently seen a therapist who suggested to her that she might solve many of her problems by "dressing more like a woman." She was visibly upset as she told me this, with tears streaming down her cheeks, and she said that she went home that night after her session with him, feeling worse than when she walked in.

With this community, the client sitting before you might look or sound like one gender, but truly and comfortably identify as another altogether, whether they are cisgender, trans, or somewhere in between. A good rule of thumb here is to simply never assume; rather, listen for clues in how your client speaks about themselves – i.e. what name they go by, and what gender pronouns they use. Or, if you must know for a question you are trying to build, simply ask them in a respectful way. Then, allow them to be themselves. Always keep in mind that it is more important for your clients to be comfortable in their own skin as well as in your office, than it is for you to be comfortable with their gender expression.

PREFERRED GENDER PRONOUNS

Similar to not assuming a client's gender before they tell you, it is important not to assume their gender pronouns before they tell you either. In SFBT we ask a lot of third-person and relational questions where you might use gender pronouns to describe the client sitting in front of you. A good way to know the preferred pronouns of a new client before asking such a question is to have a space on your consent form for them to identify that for themselves. It is *very* important that if you have a client who identifies as transgender or otherwise gender-fluid, you call them not just by their preferred name but also by the preferred pronouns they have identified. Sometimes it is not easy to completely forgo societal norms, and a person who looks like a male to your eyes and sounds like a male to your ears might truly be, and identify as, a woman – and vice versa. However much discipline it might sometimes take, it is incredibly important to allow your client to be who they are while in your office, and to ask questions of them in a respectful way.

PREFERRED NAME

Oftentimes, a client's legal name is not what they prefer to go by. This is certainly true of transgender folk, but also of others in the LGBT community in general. A helpful way to identify this is to have two spaces on your consent form, one for legal name and another for preferred name. Once you know it, always refer to a client by their preferred name.

In the LGBT community you will come across some unique and varying relationship dynamics. Sometimes, for example, gay men will be in a closed relationship with two other gay men, and it is important, as a solution-focused therapist, to assume that these clients know what is best for them and to ask questions about their preferred future based on the assumption that they can succeed healthily in this unique relationship dynamic.

I recently met with a lesbian couple who allowed each other to kiss other women, as long as they were honest about it and it never went further than that. Unconventional relationship dynamics are a big piece of working with this community, so simply trust that the clients you see know what is best for them and for their relationships.

THE EXTENT OF TRANSITION

With clients who identify as transgender it is important that the solution-focused therapist believes that however much or little of a transition this client wants to go through, the client knows what's best. If a trans-client does not want to take hormones or have surgery, but still identifies as trans, it is important for their clinician to respect this. Further, if they want to begin hormones one day, and the next decide that waiting a while longer is best for them at this time, we work with them as the experts in their lives throughout that process.

IF, WHEN, AND HOW TO COME OUT

In your work with the LGBT community you will come across clients who, for one reason or another, simply cannot be 'out.' Alternatively, you may see a client who knows that coming out is going to have negative ripple effects throughout their life, but who feels the need to come out anyway. Always remember that our LGBT clients know what is best for their lives. It is simply never our place to push them in one direction or another. Our job is to ask good questions, and to allow our clients to move toward their preferred future by answering them.

Putting it all into practice

The language of solution-building conversations

As noted earlier, solution-building conversations are quite different from problem-solving ones. The previously mentioned *Briefer* manual

(George et al., 2011) lists the qualities of a well-described preferred future, and I've listed these below. Their writing led me to think about the qualities of *all* of the answers that we listen for, from best hopes, to preferred future, to preferred past, to the next small steps. And subsequently I considered how we use language, as disciplined solution-focused therapists, to elicit answers with those specific qualities. So I took their amazing list, and simply described them as they were applicable to all of the answers we listen for throughout a solution-focused session; and, subsequently, I developed a list of the qualities of well-formed solution-focused questions.

The qualities of the answers that we listen for

Here are the qualities that BRIEF outlines for a well-formed preferred future. (I will be outlining and expanding upon these qualities as they come up in both the best hopes chapter and the preferred future chapter, through transcripts and stories.)

- positive: what is present rather than what is absent;
- small, concrete, and observable;
- significant to the client;
- realistic;
- recognized as involving hard work;
- interactional: affecting relationships.

(George et al., 2011, p. 12)

The qualities of well-formed solution-focused questions

So, how do we ask questions in a way that elicits such responses? Here are some qualities I've outlined of well-formed questions in an SF session:

- *Encompass solution-focused tenets and assumptions*
  From "What are your very best hopes from our work together?" to "How would you notice moving just one point higher on that scale?" every single question you see in this book will be easily tied back to some SF assumption, tenet, or principle, and some will be able to be tied back to several at once.

- *Use the client's language*
  As you read the transcripts and stories provided throughout this book you will notice that many times the therapist has just used the client's *exact* words from their previous answer to form the very next question they ask. The reason for this is that the client's language is their reality, and by respecting that and by using their words to build questions, clients are better able to connect with the question and subsequently answer in ways that are meaningful to them.

- *Only address that which the client has given them permission to ask about*

  Our clients give us permission to ask about topics, simply by bringing those topics up in session. If the client hasn't yet mentioned it, it is not our business, and therefore we assume that it is not helpful to the conversation. For example, if a client who is transgender hasn't spoken of transition via hormones or surgery, than a disciplined solution-focused clinician would not be the first to mention it in the session. Further, if a gay client hasn't yet touched on coming out, then the SF therapist neither asks about it nor otherwise addresses it.

- *Are respectful*

  Many times questions can sound respectful, but given the context are actually quite invasive and disrespectful. For example, if a transgender client brings up surgery – by saying that they hope to complete the transition they're making with a surgical procedure one day – it is certainly respectful to then ask questions around it, such as "How will you know when the day has come to take that step?" But asking, "Will you have bottom surgery?" would certainly not be a respectful a way to build on what the client has just said. A question can easily come off as nosy and invasive, and that specific information is none of our business until the client makes it so. Building on their hopes by using their language without getting into specifics that are none of our business requires great discipline, and, especially with the LGBT community, having that discipline is of the utmost importance.

- *Are tenacious*

  When you know you've just asked a good solution-focused question that both builds upon what the client has just said in a respectful and meaningful way, *and* is aimed at moving the conversation closer to the client's identified preferred future, then one of two things will happen: you will get an answer that you can build on, or you won't get an answer you can build on, maybe not even getting an answer at all. With the latter, you have a *golden* opportunity to be respectfully tenacious and quietly wait until the client answers the question, or, if it seems they have no plan to answer, simply re-ask the question in a different way. You will see examples of this throughout the book that will help you know when to stick to the question you are asking until you get a good answer, or when to assume the fault lies with the question, and abandon the question completely and move on to another.

- *Elicit details*
  Throughout this book you will see examples of questions that elicit details of the client's hopes, preferred future, next small steps, or past instances of success. Getting such details is *incredibly* important to solution-building because it aids us, and our clients, to picture exactly what is going well when things are, were, or will be, better for them. Further, the more details we get, the more likely the client is to leave the session and begin to notice those details as they occur.

The stages of a solution-building conversation

As I mentioned in the Introduction, the rest of this book is broken down, chapter-by-chapter, into tasks: five tasks of the first solution-focused conversation, followed by a chapter about the tasks involved in subsequent sessions.

Task 1: Obtaining the client's best hopes

The very first task of session number one is to obtain a destination description from the client based solely on their very best hopes from the work you will do together. As Elliott Connie (2013, p. 16) once wrote, "Establishing a best hopes for therapy is key to the therapeutic process because it establishes a direction for the rest of the conversation." Chapter 3 is devoted to explaining both why this is important, and how to successfully complete this task with an LGBT client before moving on to the next stage of the conversation.

Task 2: Connecting with and getting to know the client

In this second task of the first solution-building conversation, the therapist puts aside 'therapy' for a moment, and just asks the client some general questions about their life. These questions will elicit details about such things as work, family, where they are from, and what they like to do in their spare time.

In Chapter 4 you will learn that there is some very important work being done in this stage of therapy that will allow the clinician to ask more meaningful questions in the stages to come. This task, put in this specific place during the conversation, is another valuable piece of what Elliott Connie has contributed to solution-focused practice. Elliott wrote about doing this *after* establishing the best hopes – this part of the session had been written about previously as the very first task to complete. As you learn about this in the chapter dedicated to its use, the reasons behind doing this second, rather than first, will be explained further.

Task 3: Detailing the preferred future

Certainly the most well-known piece of SFBT, the miracle question, is fundamental to the first solution-building conversation between therapist and client. Done correctly, most of the first session is spent obtaining detail after detail of the client's preferred future, as they imagine it to be. In Chapter 5 I will go into great detail about how a good preferred future question is asked, and what techniques the solution-focused clinician can use, while obtaining details, to keep the conversation moving forward in meaningful ways.

Task 4: Scaling

Once we have a complete answer to the miracle question, it is time to introduce scaling. In the first session these scales range from zero to ten, where ten equals the miracle day as the client has just described it, and zero represents the opposite. Chapter 6 will go into detail about the importance of scaling, how to word a scaling question, and the different types of scales you can utilize with your LGBT clients.

Task 5: Compliments and feedback

After scaling, the solution-focused therapist might take a brief break to conceptualize their thoughts and then let the client know what they've learned about their strengths, resources, and ability to move toward their identified preferred future throughout this first conversation. In Chapter 7 you will learn about the importance of this piece of the session, and see examples – through transcripts and stories – of how to successfully accomplish this task with an LGBT client.

"What's been better?" Highlighting progress in subsequent sessions

This is the very first stage of every subsequent session that a solution-focused clinician has with their clients. Highlighting the progress from the previous days and weeks is key to continuing the solution-building process. In Chapter 8 you will read examples of how this is done, and learn how to tenaciously but respectfully seek this important information from your clients. The rest of this chapter will reiterate skills already gone over in great detail in previous chapters, such as scaling and the continuation of future-focused conversations.

Conclusion

Sometimes people talk about the "spirit" of SFBT, and I think that a pure belief in these tenets, principles, and assumptions is what they mean by this. Throughout the rest of this book, and as you read each chapter dedicated to the task at hand, you will get an opportunity to see how these solution-focused tenets, assumptions, and understandings look in *my* sessions with LGBT clients, and you'll see many of the techniques and questions that have been developed *so far* in correlation with them. You'll read transcripts and stories about my work, and with every utterance my hope is that you will see how it was guided by the tenets and principles I have outlined here. However, if you only take one thing from this entire book, I hope it would be that solution-focused brief therapy is *not* about those specific techniques or rote questions; rather it is about some *very* strict assumptions about people and what is helpful in therapy. The techniques and questions I use throughout this book are simply what I've found works best for me in compliance with those assumptions. In fact, I believe that if you stopped reading here, and went about your practice adhering stubbornly to the assumptions, tenets, and principles outlined in this chapter, never once wavering, you would be doing solution-focused brief therapy, whatever questions came.

3 The hopeful LGBT client

Eliciting a destination description

Let your hopes, not your hurts, shape your future.
(Robert Schuller, 1983)

We've already established that one of the core assumptions held by a solution-focused therapist is that clients come to us with hope. Heather Fiske (2005, p. 4) points out that "Just entering the therapeutic conversation, at any level, seems to us to be a statement of hopefulness." This assumption allows the very first question that we ask to be aimed squarely at identifying that hope from the work to be done in therapy. This hope is elicited by asking some version of this very simple question: "What are your very best hopes from our work together?"

One of the things I love about starting out in this way is that it puts clients in the driver's seat immediately, from the very utterances of the session. That way the client gets to determine where the conversation will be aimed, and the therapist learns *immediately* what they should be asking questions about.

I was introduced to what is known as the "best hopes" question during graduate school. In my practicum, Dr Peter Lehmann taught about SFBT using the previously mentioned manual by the London-based therapy and training center called BRIEF. I remember sitting with my fellow interns, Dr Lehmann, and another solution-focused therapist and supervisor named Tom Lee, engulfed in a conversation based on the word "from" versus the word "for." As you can see, the best hopes question, as written above, uses the word "from." I remember learning that day that BRIEF teaches it that way quite deliberately. In their manual, it is explained that the word "from" is more useful because it "implies that what is important is to know what differences are being looked for outside of the therapy"; while "for", "perhaps invites the client to give an agenda of problems to be discussed in the meeting" (George et al., 2011, p. 9). And the SF therapist wants to know right off the bat what the client is hoping their life will look like as a result of successful therapy, and therefore the wording is "from." I felt an understanding sweep over me that afternoon that language is *incredibly* important in this therapy model, and that even the slightest difference in our words can completely shift the direction in which the conversation moves. This was an important lesson that I would continue learning throughout my time as a student, and later as a practitioner.

A therapist has a couple of motivations for seeking the client's hopes right off the bat, in-session. The first is to invite the client to immediately be thinking of the desired outcome of therapy (Iveson, George, and Ratner, 2012a). And on the flip side of that reason, the answer to this question tells us, as their hired 'helper,' exactly what *we* should be aiming our questions towards for the rest of our time in-session together. Thus, it is important to both parties.

As I was considering the logic behind eliciting the client's hopes from therapy, I realized that one of the most common questions that adults ask the kids in their lives can be classified as a kind of best hopes question. "What do you want to be when you grow up?" is something that just about every well-meaning adult asks the beloved children in their lives. From teachers, to parents, to aunts, uncles, and grandparents, we all ask this question, and were likely asked it by the adults in our lives when we were young. And when you think about it, we ask it for some very logical reasons. We are encouraging these kiddos to think about their preferred future, so that they can begin doing things to prepare effectively for it as early as possible. But more than this, we are likely hoping to find some things that *we* can do to help them along the way to that career becoming a reality, such as putting them in the right extra-curricular activities, getting them into the right schools, having them practice their craft, or read books related to their hoped-for career. This question is key to helping both child and their loved ones to begin moving towards a future where that career is a reality, very much as asking "what are your best hopes from our work together?" is key to helping the participants in the therapeutic process move towards a useful conversation in therapy.

Best hopes as a contract

In their book *Brief Coaching*, the authors call this piece of the therapeutic conversation "establishing a contract" (Iveson et al., 2012a). This process of eliciting hope from clients allows both the client and the practitioner to develop an understanding of where the conversation ahead will lead, and it serves as a verbal contract about what will follow – a contract wherein the therapist agrees to ask questions about their client's hopes from therapy, and the client agrees to answer such questions.

In order to effectively contract, the therapist needs to first have a useful answer to the best hopes question, one that has the qualities that are outlined a bit later in this chapter; and subsequently, the therapist needs to summarize what was just agreed upon, making certain that they have correctly heard and understood what the client hopes for, so that both parties are consciously on the same page. You'll see in the coming transcripts, under the heading "Contracting" that this last piece of the first task is done very specifically, using the client's language to make sure that they are in agreement about where the conversation will be aimed.

Once the clinician knows that they have a good answer and have subsequently contracted with the client, the task of establishing a destination is complete and it's time to move on to the next piece of the conversation.

So, how do you know you have a good answer to contract with?

Qualities of a well-formed best hopes description

Knowing how to effectively elicit a useful answer to the best hopes question, and knowing when the question has been answered in full, and that the client is ready to contract, is a skill that takes some practice to hone. In order to truly get a sense of what the client hopes for from therapy, the solution-focused therapist has to be listening for, and building upon, answers that contain some of the qualities previously outlined in Chapter 2, while respectfully working around or brushing aside the answers that don't have those qualities. The goal here is to develop a clear but broad idea of the destination of the therapeutic conversation; as well as to identify specific and meaningful descriptors that can be used by the practitioner when later eliciting details of the clients' preferred future.

The presence of something, rather than the absence of something

The initial answer that the client gives to the question, "What are your very best hopes from our work together?" might be something like, "To not be depressed anymore." The novice solution-focused practitioner might simply accept this answer, or even assume that this client must then want to be happy, and move forward with that assumption in tow, asking about the presence of happiness in this client's life. However, the more seasoned practitioner knows that 'to not be depressed' does not meet the necessary qualifications of a best hopes description. Knowing that the client does *not* want to be depressed anymore does not provide information about what they *do* want. The opposite of depression, for example, might be happiness to Jane, but it might be confidence to Julie, or peace to Justin. I was recently conducting a training session at a local university where I asked five of the participants to think for a second about the absence of sadness, and what was present for them when sadness was removed. They each thought about their answer, then gave five very different answers: "peace," "calm," "a sense of excitement," "full of positive energy," and "refreshed" were the five responses given.

The lesson here is that a therapist should never assume they know what it means to their client to "not be depressed anymore" or to "not" be anything anymore. This is another lesson on the importance of retaining a blank slate, for every single client that you see; and when possible let them be the one who introduces the words and descriptions that they hope for.

When a client says that they don't want to feel depressed anymore, the therapist can ask a simple question that (a) keeps the client in the driver's seat, (b) makes no assumptions about what 'not depressed' means to that particular client, and (c) elicits the presence of something other just than the absence of depression. The next question an SF therapist might ask might be something like, "OK, you'd hope to not feel depressed, what would you like to feel instead?" The practitioner must then be respectfully tenacious in maintaining focus on what their client wants, until it becomes clear what would be present as a result of their successful work together, rather than what would be absent.

This ability to be respectfully tenacious is *incredibly* important when a client has a hard time describing or putting words to what they hope for. Going back to the best hopes question that we all ask the children in our lives, if one of my beloved nieces or nephews answered, "What do you want to be when you grow up?" by saying something like "I definitely don't want to be a teacher," I would quite simply do what I imagine any other well-meaning aunt would do and say something like, "OK, not a teacher. So what *do* you want to be?" And just as one would be tenacious in asking this kiddo what they wanted to be until they indicated to us the presence of some career or interest, so we can do with our clients.

Here are some other questions you can ask when the client's first answer is to 'not' be something.

- "OK, and when you're not feeling depressed, what are you feeling instead?"
- "And what would you like to replace that depression?"
- "And when the depression is gone, what will be there instead?"

Small, concrete, and observable

When we're talking about a best hopes description, we certainly aren't looking for things as small and detailed as the preferred future description to come. However, we do need an answer that is small and concrete enough for us to build on. A bit later in this chapter you will read a transcript of a client named April. In it you'll notice that her first answer to the best hopes question is something pretty big. Her answer is one that is quite common with the LGBT community. She states that she wants to gain an "understanding" of what is going on with her, and even though that fits the description of the presence of something, I wanted a few more observable details about that, and I was wondering what she was hoping for the impact of that understanding to be. So I asked April, "If this understanding were to increase for you, how would you notice?" This had the potential to elicit the smaller and more concrete answer of self-acceptance, comfort, and feelings of elation such that she could move forward with confidence.

One of the ways that I measure whether or not the best hopes description is small and concrete enough is by asking myself if the exact words that the client has used are sufficient for me to ask a meaningful and detailed preferred future question later in the session. As you'll see in Chapter 5, I was able to use those *exact* descriptors when I asked April to detail how her life might look different with the presence of understanding, acceptance, comfort, and elation. In order to build the conversation in an observable, meaningful, and very detailed way, the solution-focused therapist must help the client move from a broad answer to one that is more specific so that the conversation ahead can continue to elicit important and meaningfully descriptive details about the preferred future they hope to move towards.

Significant to the client

In their book *Brief Coaching* (Iveson et al., 2012a, p. 34), the authors write that the solution-focused approach "has no way of knowing how people should be, no way of determining what the client should be working towards." They are pointing out that this best hopes description must come from the client themselves, and nobody else. No matter how the client comes to us, we assume that they have some hope from our work together, and our task is to elicit that hope – however long it might take.

Sometimes the answer to "What are your best hopes from our work together?" is something about somebody else in the client's life. For example, I partner with a local children's hospital to work with children and teenagers who identify as transgender, and, as I specified in Chapter 1, unlike their adult counterparts, in order for them to receive any sort of medical interventions from the doctors there – such as puberty blockers or HRT – they must (in most cases) be 16 years of age and/or (for puberty blockers with younger teens) attend counseling sessions for at least six months prior to the counselor writing a letter of support for that medical intervention. Some of these kids don't really feel the need for therapy, but are willing and motivated to attend sessions in order to begin their transition. And quite often their parents are very much on board with the six-month therapy requirement, since they want their kids to move slowly so as to ensure they are doing what is really best in making these very big medical changes. So when I ask these kids about their best hopes, the answer might come in many forms, such as, "I don't know," or "I have to be here, but I don't think I need to be," or "I want to transition, but they say I have to come here first so that you can write a letter telling them to let me." Such answers can feel a little bit daunting to a therapist just starting out with this approach, or this community. However, when one remembers that there must be some motivation within these clients, the practitioner can discover some very effective ways to elicit an effective answer that is significant to the client themselves rather than just to their loved ones or their doctors.

By way of an illustration of one way to address this situation, here is a transcript with a 15-year-old who goes by the name Josh, and who identifies as a transgender boy:

Therapist: So, what are your very best hopes from our work together?
Josh: I don't know.
Therapist: Sure. If our conversations together turned out to be useful for you, how might you notice?
Josh: I don't know. I'm not the one who wanted to come here.
Therapist: Hmm. OK. Whose idea was it for you to come here?
Josh: My parents and the doctors said I have to come to counseling for a while before I would be able to get on testosterone.
Therapist: I see. OK, Well I'm going to ask your parents about their hopes here in just a little while, but before I do, what do you imagine they would like to notice happening with you, that would let them know that you were ready to begin testosterone?
Josh: They said they want me to be sure that this path is what's right for me, but I already know it is.
Therapist: Ah hah...so how do you imagine they would notice, before even getting on testosterone, that this path really is what's right for you?
Josh: I would be happier I think. I was really depressed before I told them about this, like it was really bad before. I was in my room all the time and even thinking of suicide. But I'm not anymore, because I know I'm getting closer to doing something about it, and I think they see that. I think that would be the big thing.
Therapist: OK, so if this happiness that sounds like it's already showing itself continued to grow for you, how would they notice?
Josh: I would be out more at home, and hanging out with friends more, and I'd probably be nicer to everyone, especially my little brother, he keeps calling me Jessica...and it makes me mad.
Therapist: And when that happens, when you're out more at home, being more social with friends and being nicer to everyone, even your little brother, how might your parents let you know they noticed this increased happiness in you?

Josh: They might let me get a binder! I've been asking for one for a few
weeks. And they'd finally tell the rest of the family about it, so that
I can be myself when I'm at grandma's house or hanging out with my
aunt and cousin, rather than still being Jessica. That's when I'll know
they think this is right too.

Therapist [Contracting]: So, if our sessions here lead to you continuing
to feel happy, being out more at home, being nicer to everyone, and
being more social with your friends, such that your folks knew you
were on the right path and ready to begin HRT, and were helping you
to come out to the rest of your family, and even getting you a binder,
you would feel like coming here was helpful?

Josh: Yeah, definitely.

Realistic

Clients sometimes describe their hopes in seemingly unrealistic ways.
A gay client may say that they hope to change their sexuality, for example.
When unrealistic hopes come up, as clinicians we have the responsibility
to ask the right questions to elicit more realistic hopes from our clients.
In *Briefer* (George et al., p. 10), it is explained, "If we trust the client's
answer will always have a realistic or legitimate part however 'unrealistic',
it helps the therapist try to find out what the serious part is." And in
the book *Creating Positive Futures* (Duncan, Ghul, and Mousley, 2007,
p. 17), Rayya Ghul eloquently points out that, "What is useful about
answers to this and similar questions is how the client thinks having their
answer come true will change their life."

I think of this as the desired impact of the unrealistic hope. A client
who says that they wish not to be gay anymore, for example, provides
an opportunity for the solution-focused clinician to respectfully dig a
bit with questions around the impact of that hope – a question such as,
"OK, if you could change your sexuality, what impact would that have
on your life?" or "What difference would that make, to no longer be
gay?" And within *those* answers are bound to be some realistic hopes,
such as increased confidence, improved relationships with loved ones,
or feeling calmer or happier. And although we cannot change someone's
sexuality or gender identity – just as we cannot bring the dead back to
life, or reunite a teen's divorced parents – those other more specific hopes
can certainly be achieved through a helpful conversation.

In 2014 I participated in a training session conducted by the aforementioned Rayya Ghul, a solution-focused occupational therapist,
trainer, and author, in which she addressed this issue by asking the
attendees, "Who here would like to win the lottery?" Of course we all
raised our hands, and she then asked each of us individually, "What
difference would that make for you?" to which we each gave very different answers. "I'd be able to pay off my debt, and feel free from that

burden," "I'd put my nieces and nephews through college, and breathe easy knowing that I could help them stay on the right path," and "I'd build a house for my son and his family, so that we could be closer and improve our relationships with each other." Our answers came quickly and each one was specific to our individual, and very realistic, best hopes for our lives.

When our clients answer the best hopes question with something unrealistic, we can always remember that they came to us with realistic hope, and thus, our task is to help them to identify that hope by digging a bit further with a question like, "What difference would that make?" or simply, "What else?" until their answer comes in a more realistic form.

When the client says "I don't know"

One of the most common answers to the best hopes question is "I don't know." I once heard Elliott say something quite brilliant about this answer in one of his trainings. He said that "I don't know" typically means one of two things: it either translates to "That's a *really* good question, and I need a second to think about it," or "That was the wrong question to ask me. Try again" (personal communication, 2011). One of the ways to tell which one the client might mean is how they say it, and another is to sit quietly for a minute and see if they keep going. If they say "I don't know," and it sounds a little bit like "Hmmm…let me think about that," that's a good signal that they just need a few seconds; if they say "I don't know" as a more definitive statement, maybe they are even looking you in the eye with a blank stare after they say it, that is a signal that you need to find another way to ask that question – in which case there are a few things you can do to ask the question differently.

Here are some options for rewording the best hopes question, if it doesn't translate well the first time you ask it.

- "What would you like to notice happening in your life as a result of our successful work together?"
- "How are you hoping your life will look different after our successful work together?"
- "If our work turned out to be useful for you, how might you notice?"

Transcript: April's hope

April is a 28-year-old who, I learned through her first email to me, had only recently begun to identify as a transgender female. She came in to see me early in the summer of 2014, and after she had filled out my consent form we shook hands in the lobby and introduced ourselves.

This transcript starts immediately upon April entering my office and sitting down.

Therapist (T): So, how would you describe your very best hopes from our work together?

April: Um, I guess really it would just be to sort of flesh out, better understand what this is, maybe connecting it to my past, just getting a better overall understanding. And then as I mentioned, you know, possibly towards the end after we kind of flesh things out, possibly getting the letter and going to a doctor, and maybe just, I would like to start with just a low dose of HRT to see how it would make me feel emotionally and psychologically, I guess that would be my overall end goal, just to kind of understand this, and just, honestly too, just to discuss it openly, with someone, where I know I'm not going to be judged.

T: OK.

April: So um yeah, that's my goal.

T: OK, so if this understanding were to increase for you, in a way that was helpful, how would you notice? What would you notice happening in your life that would let you know that understanding was coming?

April: [Pause] I think that would just be my overall emotional state regarding it all. Um, and I guess my own psychological understanding of it. I've already become quite more comfortable, even after just admitting it to myself, so maybe having further elation along that route. For example when I first thought that maybe this was like a real thing and all these feelings weren't just like some sort of fetish or something like that, you know, where it's in a non-sexual way. I was just like "wow" and this wave kind of came over me. And that was only very recently, like maybe a month or two ago, and it felt very, very good. So I guess just encountering further emotions along that point to where I'm not resisting against that, would be considered my further understanding of it.

T: OK, so more acceptance?

April: Yes absolutely.

T: Comfort, and you said elation?

April: Yes, there definitely was like a wave there, I was just like "whoa, maybe this is real," and something that I can do and pursue because I want to. Because it's always been there, I've just always ignored it, or repressed it, and the feelings have never gone away in 28 years.

T: OK, so being able to move forward.

April: Absolutely.

T: And continue to be comfortable, and experience that...

April: Just in my own skin, just being able to be comfortable in that

T: OK. Anything else you'd like to have happen as a result of our work together?

April: I think that about covers how I feel. Unless you're fishing for something, for some sort of specific...

T: Nope, nope, I just want to make sure I don't miss anything so I may always ask "what else" just in case.

April: No, absolutely.

T [Contracting]: OK, so acceptance, comfort, elation, and moving forward in a way that's right for you, if you left here and noticed those things happening you would know that our work together had been successful?

April: Absolutely!

Selective listening

With April's initial answer, you'll notice that I ignored a couple of her described hopes. She said she wanted to "connect it to her past," so that she could get a better understanding. And I selected the understanding piece, while dropping the connecting it to her past piece, very much on purpose. I knew that having a conversation connecting all of this to her past was very unlikely to happen in this initial solution-focused conversation, so I anchored on the understanding. She was very much OK with that as evidenced by her continued answering, and we moved forward together from there. She also mentioned later down the line getting a letter for HRT, and that "later down the line" specification let me know that we could leave that hope there for a while so that we could address the more immediate hopes of understanding, etc.

Knowing what to pick up and carry further, and what to drop altogether or leave for later sessions, comes easier and easier the more a practitioner does it in-session or practices it with colleagues.

Conclusion

Eliciting hope is the very first layer of an effective solution-building conversation. It puts the clients into the driver's seat from the very first question you ask, which can make it much easier to keep them there as the conversation continues. It specifies the direction of the coming therapeutic conversation, and acts as a contract between client and therapist. Once this piece is completed successfully, the next task can begin.

4 Connecting with and getting to know your LGBT client

> When we tackle obstacles, we find hidden reserves of courage and resilience we did not know we had. And it is only when we are faced with failure that we realize that these resources were always there within us. We only need to find them and move on with our lives.
>
> (A.P.J. Abdul Kalam, 2013)

Once the clinician has a good idea of their client's best hopes from therapy, the task of connecting with the client can begin. This is important for several reasons: it often immediately releases any tension in the room created by nerves or stressors that the client came into therapy with. It also provides the clinician with an opportunity to gain insight into this client's, couple's, or family's strengths, resources, and values, and as Steve de Shazer (2007, p. 74) points out in *More Than Miracles*, "Once we've established that the client has skills, abilities, knowledge that helps him make it through each day, then these skills, abilities, etc. can be reasonably used to build a solution." Further, it provides an opportunity for the client to ask the clinician questions that can further their comfort with them as their therapist, and it allows the therapist and the client to both get to know and like each other before delving into the next phase of the conversation. I have learned that with the LGBT community, this connection, or lack thereof, can sometimes make the difference between success and failure in therapy.

Origins of connecting: problem-free talk

Historically, this part of the session has come first – before establishing a direction for therapy – and it has commonly been labeled as "problem-free talk." However, as a student learning this approach, the term always confused me, because in my mind all of SFBT could be considered "problem-free talk," and I wasn't quite sure how other pieces of an SF conversation were anything other than problem-free. So when I thought about this piece of the conversation, in my mind I always labeled it as 'connecting with and getting to know the client,' and have described it as such ever since. In his book, Elliott Connie (2013) calls the chapter corresponding to this part of the conversation "connecting with the couple," and naturally, I have followed suit with the title of this chapter. Though whatever you choose to call it, this piece is incredibly important to the solution-building conversation, and this is especially true with LGBT clients.

Connecting after establishing best hopes

Connie was the originator of putting this connecting part of the conversation *after* eliciting a best hopes description, rather than before – as it had historically been done. He explained to me one afternoon that he did this because he wanted clients to know immediately that he was 'getting down to business,' which seemed to help this connecting piece go more smoothly (personal communication, 2013). Once again, I thought I would experiment with the idea, and found success, so I have kept it in this place in my work as well.

Listening with a constructive ear

In their book *Interviewing for Solutions* (2008), Peter De Jong and Insoo Kim Berg write about this beginning stage of getting to know a client: "Often, in answering these questions, clients begin to reveal what and who are important to them, as well as some areas of strength" (p. 53). This piece of the solution-focused conversation looks very casual, but in fact takes a lot of discipline and skill on behalf of the clinician. Eve Lipchik (2002, p. 153) described the skill used here as listening with a "constructive ear," and to some clinicians this may come quite naturally – though to others it can take quite a bit of practice. I remember attending a training session conducted by a solution-focused practitioner named Dr Sara Smock Jordon, in which the attendees were invited to do an exercise that highlighted this skill perfectly.

Everyone in the session got into pairs, and one partner complained to the other about something annoying in their life for three full minutes. The other partner was directed to sit quietly, not saying a word, but listening for evidence of their partner's strengths, values, skills, and resources. Then we switched off, and in the end we spent a few minutes telling our partner what we had learned about their values, resources, and strengths in the time that they had spent ranting and complaining. I learned that day that you can gain a *lot* of insight into what's important to someone as you listen to them complain for a while. Listening with a constructive ear caused me to hear my partner complain about her kid's school and her teacher (who, quite honestly sounded pretty awful to me), and realize just how lucky this kid was to have a mother who was so invested in her daughter's education and well-being. And when she listened to me complain about a colleague I was having trouble with at the time, she pointed out that I seemed to be someone who cared a lot about doing good work and serving the families we worked with at a very high level. I was shocked that she took that from what I said, but when she explained why she thought what she did, I couldn't argue: she was absolutely right.

The constructive ear and coming-out stories

Often, when an LGBT client begins to answer these questions about areas of their life outside the one that they came to address, they will tell their personal coming-out story. This offers an incredibly useful opportunity to listen with a constructive ear. Within every coming-out story an LGBT person might tell, is rich evidence of that person's strengths, abilities, resources, and hopes – and especially so in the toughest of stories you might hear. And as BRIEF once pointed out, "The greater the problems a person has survived the more rich the hidden history of achievement and possibility is likely to be" (Iveson, George, and Ratner, 2012b, p. 2).

I will highlight what I mean here with a story of a couple I saw a few years ago.

Peter and David

I met with this middle-aged gay couple for the first time in the spring of 2012. When they came in they were on the brink of separation – just a few days before their 15-year anniversary – and they were absolutely desperate for help. As I was getting to know them in the first session I asked about their families and the people who were most important to them. Peter mentioned his mother and the difficult time he'd had after he came out to her. He went on to explain that a little over 21 years earlier he had told his mother, who he was incredibly close to, that he was gay, and that he hadn't seen her since. He said that his mother had become so upset by the news of her only son being gay that she responded by completely disowning him and shutting him out of her life completely. Peter was absolutely heartbroken by his mothers's reaction. He had suspected that she wouldn't like his revelation, but had hoped that she would still choose to remain an important part of his life.

For the next decade Peter never gave up hope that his mother would finally come around and re-establish a relationship with him. He reached out to her every few months, on her birthday and holidays with phone calls and thoughtful cards, but every single time that his mother answered the phone she'd hang up just as soon as she heard his voice; and with every card he sent, she sent them back unopened, always with the same note scribbled on them, "return to sender, I don't have a son."

But Peter never gave up. He kept sending loving cards, and attempting to call his mother several times a year until one day, in 2002, more than ten years later, his mother didn't hang up the phone. Fast-forward to 2012, and Peter was planning a visit with his then quite old and ailing mother for the first time since 1991.

I remember hearing this heartbreaking story and feeling incredibly impressed with Peter and his lovingly stubborn tenacity throughout those difficult years. I asked him what it was that he had within himself, what he would call that trait that kept him from giving up for so long, when for ten agonizing years his mother stubbornly refused to budge. He sat for a while pondering my question, and finally he said, "The Bible says to honor your father and mother, I was just being obedient." After I picked my jaw up off the floor, I went on to ask Peter how that honor and respectful persistence that he so clearly and quite stubbornly lived his life by, might be playing a part in keeping his current relationship together. As both he and his husband thought about that, they became a bit emotional, and began to list ways that they thought that the honor and respect that Peter exhibited with his mother might be showing up in their relationship to keep it lasting as long as it had, even through their recent troubles.

As a therapist using SFBT and listening to Peter's story with a constructive ear, I simply directed my curiosity away from problem- or diagnostic-talk and toward Peter's strengths and resources and the 'how' and 'why' of those showing up as they did. Suddenly Peter became a cooperative partner in describing what strengths he had and how those unique strengths were playing a part in keeping his relationship together. His partner also became a willing participant in this conversation that turned a coming-out story smoothly into a story about a relationship that had survived an incredibly difficult time because of those very strengths and values.

Without exception, ingrained in all of these stories is specific evidence of that client's values, strengths, and resources. Therefore, every single coming-out story that comes up in a solution-focused conversation offers this very same opportunity to elicit them for application to that client's preferred future.

Allowing the client an opportunity to get to know you

Taking a few minutes to get to know the client is important so that you can gather some good information from them about who they are, what they do, what's important to them, and what they are good at. But after you've done that, it is just as important to allow them to get to know you a bit as well.

I first started offering clients this opportunity in 2011, after a conversation with Elliott Connie revealed that he offers every client he sees this opportunity. I asked him why he did that; I had always learned in my advanced clinical classes and in the agencies I worked in to never, ever, self-disclose to clients – so his doing this seemed a bit counterintuitive to me. He said that he wasn't sure why he started to do it, but that he believed it was only fair, since we ask so many questions of our clients. He also said that he had never yet been asked an invasive question that he wasn't comfortable answering, but that he had got some positive feedback from clients about this habit – so he kept doing it. At that point I started to experiment a bit with letting my clients get to know me, and what I found in relation to my LGBT clients is that it can make a big difference.

When I first started to experiment with it, I'll admit that it felt a little bit uncomfortable. I had always learned that self-disclosure can blur boundaries and turn the tables on the therapist. But what I've learned in the years that I've been working in this way is that clients typically don't ask inappropriate questions when given a respectful opportunity to be inquisitive about their therapist. What they *do* ask is what they need to know to feel completely comfortable that you are the right therapist for them. And self-disclosing by answering these kinds of questions is very different from blurring boundaries by detailing your life difficulties and struggles in a way that would change the nature of the relationship between you and your client. Of course doing the latter would *never* be advised. But short of taking these answers that far, I would always encourage therapists to offer their LGBT clients this opportunity, and notice the difference it makes in your ability to connect throughout the rest of the session. And if a client does ask something that you aren't comfortable answering, you can simply let them know, and tell them that they don't have to answer any questions you ask them either, if they aren't comfortable doing so.

The impact of this with LGBT clients

Recalling the lesbian couple I referenced in Chapter 2, when I asked them what they wanted to know about me, one partner – who was quite masculine but very much identified as female – asked me if I had ever met a woman who looked like her. She sighed and physically relaxed when I let her know that I had personally and professionally met women who expressed their gender similarly to her. However, if I had not given her the opportunity to ask me that question, she might have felt uncomfortable throughout our entire session and that discomfort might have clouded her ability to be fully present as we went through the rest of our conversation, adversely affecting the whole session.

Looking at the transcript below, when I ask April what she wanted to know about me, her very first question is what my experience was in seeing people in her situation. I knew at the time that what she was referring to was her unique gender expression. Those questions asked over and over again from my LGBT clients are *exactly* why I always ask if there's anything they want to know about me. So many times clients in this community just want to know if the person that they have hired to help them is familiar and comfortable with their community, and thus comfortable with them as they sit in our office.

Sometimes, clients might use this opportunity to continue to break the ice with you. I've had clients ask me all sorts of questions at this point in the session. Questions like where I'm from, whether or not I'm gay, how long I've worked in private practice, if I'm in a relationship and for how long, even seemingly silly things like one client who asked me if the way my hair was graying was natural or dyed that way, or another couple who were new to town and asked me if I knew any good places to go kayaking in the area. And without fail, no matter the question, after I answer honestly, everything in the room seems to get more comfortable.

Just a few days before sitting here and writing this, I had the mother of a 14-year-old transgender male thank me at the end of our session together for allowing her and her son to ask me questions. She said she was very comfortable with me as her son's therapist simply because I offered them the option to ask me about my life and experience before jumping in and asking them all about theirs.

What about the straight clinician?

I was leading a training session recently and one of the participants asked me whether I thought straight clinicians would be successful working with LGBT clients. She seemed concerned that if her clients asked her if she was gay, and she said "no," it would hinder their ability to be comfortable with her. My response to that is that I don't know if it would or not; that would depend on several things, not the least of which is the client's opinion on that matter. But offering them the opportunity to ask might then offer them the opportunity to continue getting to know more about you and your thoughts on those matters, and thus be more comfortable in your presence. I remember when I used to work with families in an agency setting, often parents would want to know if I had any kids, and when I told them honestly that I didn't they would move on to other questions about my experience – the answers to which helped them to be more comfortable with me as their 'helper.'

Connecting with April

In the transcript below, you will read exactly how I completed this task with April.

T: OK, I wanna get to know you a bit outside of all of this. [Moving notes to the desk.]

C: OK.

T: And give you an opportunity to get to know me, if you'd like.

C: Absolutely.

T: So, where are you from originally?

C: Nevada.

T: Nevada, where in Nevada?

C: West Nevada, so I was born and raised there, and I moved when I was 19. I was experiencing massive depression and I had some sort of weird medical hiccup where I just couldn't eat anymore. My stepdad and I tried to figure out what was going on, and slowly weaned me back to food starting with some soup and rice until I could eat regularly again.

T: Wow.

C: And after that I basically just felt I needed a change in my life, so my father was from Texas, and we just decided that it would be a good thing if I moved out here, and it really was. So I moved out here and went to school and lived rent-free which was nice. And that's kind of how I ended up here.

T: Which school did you go to?

C: I went to a college in Amarillo, you might find some info about it but they shut down their entire Texas operation actually. Which is not great to tell to employers.

T: [Laughs.]

C: But I don't even have to mention it; I'm a few years into my career now. I'm a graphic designer.

T: That's what I was getting ready to ask...

C: Absolutely, I actually just got a new job today.

T: Congratulations!

C: Thank you. I was laid off my last job at the end of March. I had wanted to leave. I had been there for three and a half years, I was their only in-house designer, so I learned a lot, got what I could, but they were shutting down their office, so they gave me a severance and now I do contract work here and there. But I just landed a job today for good pay with benefits, which is nice. It's at an ad agency, which is what I wanted to move into. Before I was by myself at work, but now I'll be part of a team which is nice, I was alone at the other job, I'm good on my own but three and a half years of that got tiring.

T: So you're good at the graphic design bit?

C: Yeah I believe so.

T: What do you think makes you good at that?

C: My creativity. Um, I got into graphic design when I was young, 13 or 14...and I discovered it and got myself a copy of Photoshop, downloaded it, and started tinkering around. So I basically taught myself until I went to school. Making interesting and weird pictures out of multiple pictures to create something new. I like creating something new, and solving problems. You have to keep your cool in this field, though, because everybody's a critic about visual stimuli.

T: Ah…and how do you keep your cool?

C: Mmm…in terms of work, um…grumbling to myself a lot, just knowing that they don't know what the fuck they are talking about, but realizing that I'm an adult and this is my job so I have to figure out some way to solve the problem we're having, and that's just being an adult, in that sense, just trying to suck it up and do what I can and realize it's just work and I get off at 5pm and I could be doing retail again, and I hated that, so just realizing it's where I am and the reality of it, in a sense.

T: Nice. OK, so, how long have you lived here?

C: Six to seven years or so…

T: Alright…and who do you live with?

C: Right now I'm with my ex-girlfriend, we just broke up like three weeks ago. Normally, "Adam" of the past would be devastated by this, losing my job, losing a relationship of two and a half years, she was the second woman I've ever slept with, and the longest relationship I've ever had, everything was great but she just grew distant. We talked about it, gave it time, talked about it again, and just decided to end it. So our lease is up in July, and with this new job I'll be able to find a place to live on my own. But right now I'm just living with her…so things are cordial, I don't hate her for it, again coming down to the reality of…"well I'm an adult, things just don't work out sometimes," so I mean I can be nice about this, I'm not really angry about it. And part of the reason too, is coming to this conclusion and having this horizon to look forward to, and be interested in, and also like I said the elation of that realization. It just kind of kept me out of any sort of slump, that those two circumstances would have led me to in the past. Which they would have, I mean, there were break-ups that took like…like…it's the worst thing in the world, like you know, like in the past.

T: Yeah.

C: But now I feel really good. And I don't think it's just because I'm like ignoring it, or repressing some sort of sadness from the ending of that relationship. I look at it as just a new horizon in my life. Part of when I think about, can I do this transition, is like I'm already 28, like I've missed my twenties why didn't I think of this sooner. But then I think, I'm almost 30, and 30 is the new 20 and I think this will be awesome, and I can continue to live my life in a positive way, instead of thinking negatively and continuing to push these feelings aside.

T: OK, huh, OK, so…

C: I believe I've grown up, as a person.

T: Yeah.

C: 'Cause if we'd of had these sessions for years, the person sitting right here would be *completely* different than I was in the past. I think part of that is just growing up and realizing you can be a big person about things, and try to think logically as well, about situations, and look at more positivity in everything, instead of only the negatives. Which is what I used to do, very cynical, I still can be very cynical, before it was more in a sarcastic sort of way.

T: OK, any other important people in your life?

C: Umm, I guess two of my best friends right now, one has been my best friend since middle school, his name is Mark and he lives in California, and actually if I wasn't able to obtain a job I was going to move in with him.

T: OK.

C: I have told him all about this and he has been overwhelmingly supportive, as has his girlfriend and his roommate. So I believe still I'm going to work for about a year, and work on just some facial hair removal here, while I work and then I plan to probably move to Colorado. I've done a lot of research and they have transgender-friendly laws about the hiring process and stuff, which Texas doesn't have. And the other close person in my life would be my cousin Nathan, on my father's side. I told him recently and we hung out and he was also very supportive about this, and he's always been that way, just like "if that's what you want to do, I'm here for you." I would say in terms of key people those would be the two.

T: Nathan and Mark.

C: Yeah. I'm very close with my parents but not about this. My plan to tell them is after I've done this for a while and I have 100 percent certainty about what I'm doing, I believe they will both love me no matter what but my mother has this certain way of making me question whatever I'm doing, whether it's looking for a new apartment, or job, when I talk to her she throws out things that just make me question it. So when I tell her about this in the future, it's going to be an ultimatum, rather than anything else. My plan is email her, and tell her not to contact me until she thought about it, tell her not to call me back right away, but to talk to my stepdad who I believe would also be very supportive, he's a pretty good guy. So I'd tell her to talk to him or whoever else but to think about it before you call me back. And I'll kind of go along those lines. I'm very close with them, just not on this aspect, yet.

T: OK, anything else you'd like me to know about you? Just 'getting to know you' stuff?

C: Umm, I used to be really depressed and fight with my mom. But I was able to beat depression, and I know I beat it, because I could physically feel the difference between depressed and not depressed...and

I also have anxiety. Had full blown panic attacks in the past, but for the last decade I've been managing and working on anxiety, and it's gotten better, but again I just try to be positive and logical and I've gotten a handle on it. I guess that's it.

T: OK, is there anything you'd like to know about me, any questions that you have for me? I'm gonna continue to ask you a bunch of questions so it's only fair that you get a shot too.

C: Sure, I guess what's your experience dealing with folks in my position?

T: So, I've specialized in this community for the three years that I've been here in practice, so I've got that experience with folks all over the gender spectrum. I don't know if you have anything more specific to ask.

C: Not really.

T: OK.

C: You seem qualified.

T: [Laughs.]

C: From what I looked up online, I like that this facility was very LGBT-friendly, and focused towards that, it's what drove me to you. [Pause.] Um, I can't really think of anything else at the moment, but if I do I will certainly ask.

T: Feel free, it's only fair.

Creating the right atmosphere for connecting

You'll notice at the beginning of this task with April, I tell her that I'd like to get to know her, "outside of all of this" while simultaneously moving my notes to my desk as a deliberate symbol that we were about to have a very casual little chat. This is where the therapist can often see clients relax a little bit, almost like a physical "Phew." Often that transition is accompanied by a sigh from the client, a smile, and maybe even adjusting a bit in their seat to get more comfortable. Everyone has a reference point for 'get to know you' talk, so clients are typically quite comfortable as soon as this part of the session begins. They have no idea that you are actually about to work very hard as they answer your seemingly innocent questions.

I also give April a tip-off that I'm going to let her get to know me a bit as well. This statement is a foreshadowing of what will come after I have got to know her a bit. I say it there very much on purpose – to set us both up for the question I ask towards the end of the connecting process. I asked April about where she was from, hoping to get some useful information about her family, which I certainly received. Further, I asked her about what she did for a living so that I could get a sense of what she's good at, and have some useful information on which to address focused questions in the future. I also asked her about the important people in her life, because a very big part of many solution-building conversations is asking questions from the perspective of those people in the lives of our clients. You'll notice in the dialogue that I sought specific data about important people in April's life. Those questions were quite purposeful and that information will be used at a later point in our conversation.

April's strengths, skills, resources, and values

As you can see in the dialogue with April, she revealed a whole lot of very useful information about her values, priorities, strengths, and resources. Just a few minutes into our session April has proven that historically, given an incredibly tough situation like going through a period in her young life when she literally couldn't eat for a long time due to depression, that she can call on her resources to help her to problem-solve the situation and be willing to try something very different like moving to another state in order to seek a better life. I quietly took this information in and made a mental note of it, storing it away for later use while continuing to seek more information *just* like that. Further, I learned that April is appreciative and she seems to both enjoy and be skilled at learning from her experiences. April has perspective and the strength to get through frustrations by looking for the light at the end of the tunnel and subsequently moving towards it. Another piece of information I pulled from this piece is that when April figures out what she likes and what makes her happy, she jumps in. She began learning skills related to her eventual career at an early age and stuck with it such that she was able to make a career out of it 15 years later.

It also comes out that at the time of this session April is going through a very difficult time, breaking up with a girlfriend, a situation that she said would have torn her apart before. But she's so enthralled with her own future and what it's going to look like that she is taking it quite well and working very hard to be a good person to her ex. This is further confirmation for me, as her therapist, that when April is focusing on her future and excited about what's on the horizon, she copes extremely well with otherwise incredibly difficult circumstances.

April is on this journey of self-discovery and until she knows exactly what she's discovered she has made a conscious decision to avoid muddling the situation by telling her mother – who no doubt means well, but who April knows would simply complicate the situation with questions and comments that she wants to be fully ready for before that conversation takes place. This piece of information lets me know that with April, this journey has, so far, been very well thought out and planned.

In this conversation, April gave plenty of opportunities for problem-talk to begin, and many therapists might have delved right in, asking about the complications April brings up. However, in this task our job is to simply listen with a constructive ear, making mental notes of what we learn as we keep gathering useful information. It takes great discipline and a lot of practice to avoid digging further into the problem-focused topics that clients sometimes offer up on a silver platter at this stage of the conversation. But it is important to continue listening with a constructive ear, and doing so often offers the client the opportunity to reveal to you how they are dealing successfully with those issues already.

The unintended consequence of not connecting

I remember meeting with Leigh one afternoon several years ago, and feeling throughout the session that I was just off somehow. I never really felt like I got my footing with her, and when the session was over she didn't schedule a second meeting. I felt quite troubled and decided to talk with a colleague about the session afterwards, and how off it felt. I said that I had the feeling that Leigh didn't schedule again because she didn't find our conversation very helpful. My colleague asked me to take her through the session so that we might troubleshoot what happened, and the first thing that I told her was that Leigh had come into session clearly feeling very angry about the incredibly difficult situation she was dealing with involving her ex-wife and their teenage daughter. Her relationship had abruptly ended, although she very much wanted it to continue, and her ex was now about to leave the state with their 13-year-old daughter in pursuit of a new job and a new relationship with another woman she had recently met online. Leigh was not the biological mother of their daughter and because of the laws in Texas, even though they had been together for 15 years, and got married in a state where their marriage was legal, Leigh seemed to have no legal recourse for when her ex pulled the trigger and moved out of Texas and across the country. She was understandably panic-stricken and as angry as could be; so viscerally angry, in fact, that I got completely thrown off my usual rhythm, and rushed into detailing Leigh's preferred future, without ever taking a few minutes to get to know her outside of these issues, or allowing her to get to know me.

As I went through the session with my colleague, I realized that I essentially joined Leigh's panic, and rather than stay in my comfort zone and do what I usually did – going through the first session step-by-crucial-step – I got a bit rattled and skipped this connection piece altogether. As a consequence of that, throughout the conversation – as I was attempting to get detail after detail of her preferred future – Leigh's intense anger never waned, and she had an incredibly difficult time answering the questions, no matter how long I gave her or how many different ways I asked them.

My mistake with Leigh resulted in never having a few minutes to put everything aside (including her intense emotions) and just casually getting to know each other, and so we simply never connected. I didn't give myself the opportunity to listen for evidence of who she was outside the issues she brought with her to therapy, and I did her the disservice of never allowing her to get to know me and relax a little bit in order to move from her emotional state to a calmer place where she could have a mindset conducive to answering the future-focused questions that would follow. That mistake adversely affected the rest of that session, and was, I suspect, the reason behind it not being helpful for her. I felt terrible when I realized my error, and I vowed right then and there never to make that simple mistake again. Now, no matter what emotion the client brings into therapy, I stay focused and take the time to complete this task, and a session like that has not been repeated since.

Conclusion

Although this piece of the initial solution-focused conversation can seem very casual and relaxed, you can see now that it is an incredibly important building block in the session. Really getting to know and like your client, and respectfully allowing them to get to know and like you in return, can be the difference between a successful session and an incredibly unhelpful conversation. Done correctly, this piece of the session creates the perfect atmosphere for smoothly transitioning into the task of obtaining an incredibly detailed picture of the client's preferred future – which you'll learn about in the chapter that follows.

5 The preferred future

The best way to predict your future is to create it.

(Robert Anthony, 1999)

At this point in the session you have successfully obtained a clear idea of your client's hopes from therapy as well as some useful information about their life, their loved ones, and their values, resources, and strengths. You've given them an opportunity to get to know you a bit, and things in the room are probably pretty comfortable. This is where the real work begins.

Obtaining an incredibly detailed picture of a day in which your client's best hopes have been realized is, in many respects, the very essence of solution-focused brief therapy. The most widely recognized way of obtaining this description, and the most well-known piece of solution-focused brief therapy, is the miracle question.

Origins of the miracle question

In their book *Interviewing For Solutions* (2008), Peter De Jong and Insoo Kim Berg point out that the miracle question was formulated in the middle of a very tricky session that Insoo was having with a client. She was trying to elicit details of this client's preferred future, and the client was having a hard time answering and said that, "Maybe only a miracle will help, but I suppose that's too much to expect" (p. 84). So Insoo, demonstrating incredible tenacity and respect asked, "OK, suppose a miracle happened, and the problem that brought you here is solved. What would be different about your life?" (p. 84). Thus the miracle question was born. In that same text, the authors write about the question that evolved as a result of that successful session, and it is asked as follows:

> Now, I want to ask you a strange question. Suppose that while you are sleeping tonight and the entire house is quiet, a miracle happens. The miracle is that the problem which brought you here is solved.

However, because you are sleeping, you don't know that the miracle has happened. So, when you wake up tomorrow morning, what will be different that will tell you that a miracle has happened and the problem which brought you here is solved?

(Berg and De Jong, 2008, p. 84)

The very first utterance in the miracle question posed above is incredibly important. Giving the client a kind of warning about the question soon to be asked is both acknowledging that we are about to delve into the solution-building process (a very different kind of conversation than most clients are expecting to have), and setting the client up to pay *very* close attention as the therapist and asks this question.

Another important note is the mention of the entire house being quiet. In *More than Miracles*, Yvonne Dolan points out that "Inviting a client to answer the miracle question works best if it is conveyed in an appealing comfortable way" (de Shazer et al., 2007, p. 24). Further, the more details you put into the question – describing the surroundings as the miracle occurs – the more able to put himself into the question the client seems to be. But perhaps the most important piece of the question above is that the miracle happens while the client is asleep, thus they can have no idea that it has taken place. This detail sets the client up to imagine how they will go about noticing the very specific differences once the miracle has occurred. It puts them in the driver's seat, and allows them to steer their imagination towards the description of a day that *they* see as miraculous. It also allows the client to go about discovering the miracle in real time, right there in-session as they answer the question, detail by imaginative detail. In *More than Miracles*, the authors say "the client and therapist go on a collaborative search in the client's real, everyday world to discover the signs that indicate the miracle has happened and the problems are gone" (de Shazer et al., 2007, p. 39). So the client can imagine themselves discovering this miracle, and actually *be* discovering it at the exact same time.

As you'll notice throughout the transcript and stories in the rest of the chapter, as clients detail these miracle days they describe what they will be doing, seeing, feeling, and thinking differently, and many of those details are incredibly realistic actionable descriptions, furthering their ability to leave the session and begin to create the future they have just described.

The miracle question evolved

In the aforementioned version of the miracle question, you might recognize that there was no mention of the client's best hopes, or destination descriptions. This is where I will point to the evolution of SFBT. BRIEF and the practitioners who founded it address this evolution when they say, "At BRIEF we began to rephrase the question so that instead of saying that the miracle solved problems, we said that the miracle led to the client's best hopes being achieved" (George et al., 2011, p. 19).

There are other examples of clinicians using something other than 'the problem that brought you here is solved' since the miracle question's inception. In the book *Creating Positive Futures*, Ghul offers a transcription where the therapist asked about a miracle wherein the client's life "becomes the way you would like it to be" (Duncan et al., 2007, p.18). So whether one uses the best hopes as an initial destination description, or some other form of eliciting the client's desired outcome from therapy, many practitioners now use the presence of the client's desires, rather than the absence of the problem in their wording of this question.

You'll see very specific examples of incorporating a client's best hopes into a preferred future question with LGBT clients a bit later in this chapter.

Qualities of a well-described preferred future

Most of the first session is spent getting a detailed picture of a full day in the client's preferred future, from the very moment the miracle begins – with the therapist keeping in mind the kinds of answers they are seeking, and clarifying with specific questioning throughout. The therapist builds on the very last thing that the client said and makes sure that their answers have the qualities they are looking for until they get as many details as possible. In *Interviewing for Solutions* (De Jong and Berg, 2008, p. 85), it is pointed out, "The practitioner's task is to pose a series of related questions to invite the clients to express their vision of a more satisfying future." These questions build upon the last utterance of the client, and move from one moment to the next in the miracle day that the client is describing.

Here are five of the necessary qualities of a good description of that future as they are outlined in *Briefer* (George et al., 2011), with some explanation about each one:

Small, concrete, and observable

The first thing for a practitioner to remember in order to elicit the kind of answer that is very detailed and thus, useful, is to start very small. The question asks for the very first thing the client would notice, and in asking for that the practitioner is inviting the client to start from the beginning as well as to start small. In *More than Miracles*, the authors point out

> Concrete, detailed descriptions of behavior and action constitute a virtual rehearsal of what a person wants to do in his or her life. The more detailed the description, the more vivid or 'real' the experience

becomes for the client, thereby making it easier and more natural to carry out in real life.

(de Shazer et al., 2007, p.46)

Often, though, the client might start to answer the miracle question with something they would be feeling, such as waking up and feeling 'happy.' The practitioner has an opportunity then to move from a feeling to the impact that feeling would have on their daily actions by gently probing for behavioral details of 'happy' – by asking something like, "What would be the first move you'd make, after waking up filled with this happiness?"

The authors of *More than Miracles* address another benefit of getting these small, concrete, answers from our clients when they say, "the positive feelings evoked by this behavioral descriptive process can be an invaluable source of much-needed 'courage for the journey' " (de Shazer et al., 2007, p. 46). When you are talking with an LGBT client who is on a journey of self-discovery, where coming out of the closet or physically transitioning into their true self is a piece of their preferred future, courage is the most important piece of moving forward. Sometimes a client comes into therapy seemingly unable to summon that 'much-needed courage' it will take to create the life they desire. Detailing the many positive impacts of waking up happy or confident, and living the life they hope to as a result, can create that courage and help it to grow into action after that client leaves the session.

I've seen the impact of such conversations help many LGBT clients to move forward in what they had previously identified as pretty daunting ways. I recently met with a client who was 21, and newly identified as bisexual. He had never pursued a relationship with another male, but very much wanted to gain the courage to explore that aspect of his sexuality. He was understandably nervous about this new path, but also quite eager to explore it. We spent an hour describing the version of himself that acted with courage and confidence, exploring his attraction to other men in a way that was right for him and his life. When I met with him the following week, he'd added himself to a gay dating website, one that was much more about actual dating than about simply 'hooking up,' which, he found, many gay male sites were; and he had set up a lunch date with a guy for the following day. He remarked that he left our first session feeling very brave, after describing for an hour what that courage would look and feel like once he had it, and he was able to then use that courage to begin taking steps that very night. He found that his courage stayed with him, and though he was still a bit nervous, he felt more excited than scared, and very much looked forward to really exploring this new path. I met with him three more times, and by our last session he had been dating a guy he met on that site for several weeks, and was incredibly happy with where he was.

The presence of something, rather than the absence of something

Clients will often begin listing signals around things that would be absent – such as not feeling angry anymore, or not feeling self-conscious. The therapist's job is to listen and follow their client's answer while respectfully eliciting the presence of feelings, rather than their absence. Returning to the trusted "What would you feel *instead*?" is a good way to help the answer get rolling a bit. Another good way to help nudge clients towards these kinds of descriptions is to ask them what they would be seen doing – from a third-party perspective – of either a pet, a loved one, or even a hypothetical camera, if it were following them around after this miracle occurred. For many clients the answers start to come much more quickly after a few details start the building process, and the descriptions get easier to detail with every answer they give as they learn the language of solution-building.

Significant to the client

Often when the client gives details about the preferred future, a clinician can help drive home the importance of that detail by asking something like, "Would that be different, to wake up and feel at peace?" or "And how would you know that it was the right decision, choosing to come out to your sister on this day?" Or one that I've recently used with a lesbian couple who reported not being intimate for several months prior to our first session. One of the partners said that after this miracle occurred, she'd wake up feeling at peace, and would turn and give her sleeping wife a kiss. I asked her wife, "And would that be a pleasant way for you to wake up, with such a kiss?" And, blushing, she said emphatically and humorously, "Oh yeah…I'd call into work and we'd be in bed all day!"

These kinds of emphasis questions amplify the significance of these shifts in the client's life, and can drive home the impact of doing things differently in their preferred future. This is important because applying affirmative feelings to action descriptions adds richness to the preferred future description that may otherwise be missed. Doing this can act to further increase that courage to go and create a life filled with those descriptors after they leave the session.

Realistic

If the practitioner is not careful in their wording of this miracle question, the answer might come in the form of something unrealistic. With the LGBT community, it might come in the form of an immediate physical transition, overnight, or they might hope to wake up and not be gay, bi, or trans.

The most effective way I've found to elicit a realistic answer to the miracle question is to simply insert the already-established realistic best hopes into the question, and maybe to add some qualifiers within the question itself, just to be sure it comes in realistic form. For example, in the question I ask April below, I specify that the miracle I'm asking about happens only within her, not outside of her or effecting her physically at all. I did that very much on purpose, to avoid a response such as, "I'd suddenly have the body I want," or "Texas would change its laws to protect my transition in regards to work." Adding those qualifiers helps keep the answer restricted to the already-established very realistic hopes from therapy. Another benefit of asking it with such qualifiers is that it reduces the risk of an answer coming in the form of things that may be realistic but out of the client's control – such as other people, not present in the session, changing and being better, rather than the client being at their best.

Recognized as involving hard work

When clients talk about their preferred future, quite often their initial answers are quite simple, as in they'd "just feel happy." However, when we 'feel' happy we also 'do' happy, and the details around how we individually 'do' happy contain clues to achieving and maintaining that very happiness.

I was recently talking with a client and she was describing her miracle day, and a job interview she was preparing for. She said she'd get up early, right when her alarm went off, and feel confident. I asked her what a morning full of confidence looked like for her, and she described a very disciplined morning, where she ate breakfast, showered, took time to make herself look great, ironed her clothes, and gave herself a positive pep-talk in the mirror. I commented that it must take a lot of discipline to get up early enough to do all of that – before an early morning job interview – and she responded that yes, when she's at her best she works very hard to get what she wants.

Sometimes people criticize SFBT, saying that it's too positive, seemingly feeling as though it's unrealistically so, but the client's answers are typically full of details where they are completing difficult tasks throughout their day, and in that hard work lies the secret to 'doing' the confidence or happiness they are after in the first place.

Interactional: affecting relationships

As you go through the details of the miracle day, oftentimes (and especially with couples and families), other people or even pets will come into the picture. It can quite easily be assumed that the miracle would impact the way in which the client interacts with those loved ones in their life. Further, as noted above, when a client gets stuck on a descriptor, asking what their family/friend/dog/co-worker would notice about them that would let them know something was different, can get the answers rolling again in very significant ways.

In *More than Miracles*, Dolan writes:

> Asking a question incorporating the view or reaction of someone with whom the client has a relationship anchors the therapeutic change more concretely in the client's real life, and provides a sign-post of progress that she can look at in the future when she in fact does what she is describing and the other person responds.
>
> (de Shazer et al., 2007, p. 26)

These third-person questions offer a unique opportunity to clients within the LGBT community to imagine their loved ones noticing the positive impacts of coming out of the closet, or moving forward in a new relationship, or even transitioning. Imagining such scenarios can help them to reach past the fear they might have about such revelations, and into the behavioral reality of a future in which they are being true to themselves, and experiencing positive impacts that are clearly visible to those around them. And more, it sets them up to recognize those shifts in their loved ones – maybe even before their loved ones notice it themselves.

Preferred future descriptions with LGBT clients

Scott's miracle: getting back to normal

I remember meeting with Scott for the first time in the fall of 2014. He called me on a Tuesday afternoon and left me a voicemail requesting a same-day session. That kind of phone call from a first-time client typically indicates some urgency, and when I called him back I could tell that Scott was in crisis. I had an opening that day so we scheduled a session for a few hours later.

Scott is an openly gay 32-year-old, and, having come straight from work as a nurse, he came into session still wearing his scrubs. He explained that he had been diagnosed with HIV about a month prior to our visit. Scott's life had been spiraling out of control since the diagnosis, and he was absolutely desperate for some relief. He said that for the last 30 days he had been in the worst state of his life. He had become completely obsessed with learning everything there was to know about HIV, and he was feeling out of control, depressed, and extremely anxious. He said his previously very healthy relationship was beginning to suffer, as was his job, which had always been positive and fulfilling for him, and even his friendships were beginning to fade. He was having a hard time focusing at work, a situation that he feared, if it continued, could negatively impact his patients. He was considering taking a leave of absence, but he just couldn't afford to do that at the moment.

Scott's best hopes from our work together were to get back to some sense of normalcy and control in the face of this new diagnosis, and to find the strength to accept this reality that had been thrust on him so suddenly and unexpectedly. He wanted to feel better so that he could feel excited about life, and get his relationship, career, and social life back on track.

I remember asking Scott about his preferred future very carefully. I did not want to seem more optimistic or hopeful than he was, for fear that he would think I wasn't taking his incredibly difficult situation seriously enough. I wanted to honor his feelings, and ask him about a realistic future where this diagnosis was real and taken seriously, but he was somehow able to take that control and find acceptance in the new 'normal' his life was moving towards. I remember thinking that this question needed to be asked *just* right, in such a way that I could respect the absolute difficult reality of his situation while I asked it. So I thought about it a minute before asking the following question:

> OK Scott, I've got kind of a strange question for you now, if you're ready. [Pause while Scott nodded to indicate readiness.] Imagine for a moment that we finish talking here today, and you go about your day just as you were planning to. You go home to Jeff; maybe you have dinner and play with Spike [their dog] a bit, you do whatever it is that you were planning. Eventually you get ready for bed as you typically would, and you lie down to go to sleep for the night, just as you usually do. But while you're sleeping, Scott, imagine that a miracle happens within you. Nothing about your life or diagnosis changes, nothing about Jeff or your job changes, but you are suddenly filled with the strength and ability to find acceptance and normalcy in the face of this new reality, such that you can once again be at your absolute best throughout your day tomorrow.
>
> But the trick here is, that since this miracle happened while you were asleep, you didn't feel it, so there is no way for you to know that it has occurred except to go about discovering it after you wake up tomorrow morning. What would be the very first clue that would signal something miraculous must have happened, and you were once again at your absolute best in this new reality?

As you can see with the miracle question as it is posed above, the wording was chosen quite carefully. I wanted to make it clear that this miracle was something that just happened within Scott, not to his partner or to his diagnosis, just to him and his ability to reach his previously established best hopes, overnight. Very specific information about his life was purposely chosen to craft this question, keeping him in control of defining his hopes within the details of that miracle day. Personal information about his partner, Jeff, and even their beloved dog Spike was included. I've noticed in my practice that the client seems to more easily connect to the question when these personal details are sprinkled into it, as it adds rich context to them as well as showing the client that you have been listening to the things that are important to them. Further, rather than addressing the 'problem' as I worded the question, I inserted Scott's already-specified very realistic best hopes, and the question was built around the sudden and miraculous presence of them.

When Scott answered this question he talked about waking up with that sense of excitement again, and accepting the new reality, of living with HIV – similarly to how he had accepted life as a gay man when he came out to himself. As I sought more and more details about this day, moment by moment, he talked about waking up to his alarm feeling that excitement and popping out of bed without pressing the snooze button. He detailed making coffee with his favorite creamer, playing with his dog, and laughing and joking with Jeff before going into work. He described driving into work with the windows down, feeling the wind on his face, and listening to upbeat music. At work he detailed focusing with great care on his colleagues and his patients. He has a good friend who works with him, and he talked about her noticing this miracle the moment she saw him. He described the smile on his face and the jokes and sarcasm that would be a part of his interactions once again. He gave details about making plans to go shopping with friends again. He said he would be looking forward to picking up on remodeling his house, and fantasizing dreamily in his downtime about the work to be done. Remodeling was a project he started prior to the diagnosis, but had since let go. He mentioned his friends becoming a priority again, and socializing with them in the evening and on weekends. He would have an appetite again, and so going out to dinner or for coffee would be as positive and relaxing as it used to be. He said Jeff would notice the fun and goofy Scott being back, and that he would be very pleased to have a partner to play with him like he used to. When I asked him about the difference it would make for him, to be this happy, excited, energetic, funny version of himself, he said getting back to that version of himself would help him feel more normal, and make this new diagnosis feel manageable. He compared the feeling he imagined coming along with his best self to the feeling that he got after he finally came out, and found acceptance with himself as a gay man in Texas.

When I saw Scott again just four days later, he said that after he left he immediately began experiencing the details he described in our first session, and that he already felt more normal. He wasn't exactly where he wanted to be, but he had made some significant progress in just a few days time. He was able to be totally present at work, even through an incredibly difficult day during which a patient had almost passed away and there had been conflict among his co-workers. He said he was more relaxed in all aspects of his life, and that he was feeling much better; and that it suddenly became very clear to him what had been hindering his ability to be happy.

He said that as a result of working in the medical field, he had access to journals and papers about HIV and AIDS, and that since his diagnosis he had created a habit of pouring over them in an effort to understand the disease more, and learn all about new developments and treatments. He also created a habit of looking at his medical printouts from his doctor's visits, his blood count, and other pieces of data that he needed to keep an eye on for the rest of his life, and he began to overanalyze them. He said that over the last four days he hadn't read any of that information at all, and he thought that decision must have contributed to helping things feel so much better.

In that second session he made the decision to take more control over what he looked at and when he looked at it, so that he could experience that calm, happy, and carefree version of himself more often than the anxious and depressed one he had experienced too much of in the previous month. He decided to only do any reading about his diagnosis in the morning, rather than at night before bed (which would hinder his ability to sleep well), and that he would limit himself to only doing it once a week or less when he could. This decision helped a calm wash over him, as he took control and continued to do what he thought he needed to, but only in what he now deemed as healthy doses. Scott was able to describe a very realistic preferred future and as a result of his solution-building, after session number two, he was ready to terminate therapy.

One of the most difficult things that I've ever learned about asking the miracle question is how to ask it when a client is quite clearly in crisis – as Scott was the day we met. I've made my fair share of mistakes in such situations, and the lessons I've learned have been invaluable to me. One of the biggest mistakes I would make in the early days of learning and practicing this approach was the very common rookie error of being more eager and energetic than my client. Sometimes a therapist can get away with that, and the client will join your level of energy, but with many clients – and especially with a client in crisis – it is much more likely that you will miss connecting with them and as a result not be very helpful at all.

Sharon's miracle: putting myself first

I remember meeting Sharon for the first time in the winter of 2013. Sharon was 58, and a well-respected family doctor in a neighboring city. She had recently come out to herself as a transgender woman, and the first time she came to me was the first time she spoke this truth out loud. She hoped to find the courage to begin her transition and for the first time in her life put herself first, such that she could truly move toward the person she felt she was always meant to be. Her challenges ahead were quite daunting, as her colleagues, patients, ex-wife, and teenaged daughter all only ever knew Sharon as Shawn. But she was determined to make these changes in her life and prove to herself and everyone around her that she had what it took to become herself, no matter the obstacles.

As Sharon and I went through the details of her miracle day, she described waking up at 4am to prepare for the intense workday ahead, and giving herself the time to make a warm cup of tea and sit in front of a fire in her living room, just being quiet and soaking in the peace before anyone else in the world was awake.

She described coming out emotionally and behaviorally at first, and beginning to make the shift to her more feminine self on this day, weeks before even starting to take hormones. She talked about feeding her nurturing side and having the confidence to wear pink scrubs and have hidden painted toenails at work. She described working with her head held high, rather than looking down as Shawn was used to doing, and she talked in great detail about being more social and extroverted than Shawn had ever been before. I asked Sharon what her patients would notice about her on this confident day, where she was truly connected to herself and others around her, and she detailed a doctor who made direct eye contact and went slowly as she spoke to each and every patient and family member. She talked about them noticing that she really cared about them and their situation by how much she listened and attended to their needs, regardless of how hurried she might be feeling to move on to the next task of her incredibly busy workday. She said that side of her, which she had always seen as too feminine to show before, would be allowed to take over in her professional life as a result of this miracle, and she very much imagined that both she and her patients would be all the better for it.

When I saw Sharon again a few weeks later she was quite clearly happier and more confident than when we first met. She said she did notice the difference she was able to make at work as a result of the acceptance and confidence she had gained since our first meeting, and, even though they still saw Shawn on the outside, her patients were now remarking for the first time in her career about how much they appreciated their doctor's incredible soft, thoughtful, and nurturing bedside manner. The changes she made continued to snowball over time, and today Sharon is fully transitioned and as happy and confident as she imagined herself to be on that first visit to my office.

April's transcript: the preferred future

When I asked April about her miracle, I asked her to describe the details of a miracle having happened immediately after our session ended. This dialogue was very different from dialogue after the traditional miracle question is asked, and it isn't something I do very often. The description still offered some very good details that for April proved quite meaningful.

T: OK April, I've got a strange question for you now…
C: Sure.
T: Imagine that you walk out this door today, and suddenly you're filled with that understanding of yourself, the comfort, the elation, the acceptance that you're seeking. The world doesn't change, nothing about your life changes, but you are suddenly as confident and accepting, comfortable, and understanding of yourself as you want to be, such that this horizon that you've mentioned here several times is as clear as you would like it to be. So it's a little bit of a miracle, just kind of within you.
C: Mm hmm…
T: What would be the first signal to you, after you walked out this door, even just from here to the elevator, what would be the very first signal that something miraculous must have happened, and this understanding had found you?
C: That I could mentally tell myself that it is OK to be myself, with these feelings and actually believe it, 100 percent. Now I can tell myself that, but I'm questioning it constantly, and I know that humans just question things constantly, we are a very inquisitive race, but to able to just have that moment when I could say this to myself and be like "yeah, I absolutely can. Fuck everybody else, like, what they think doesn't matter, it's what you think and what you feel." And then I'd actually ingest that, to where I would know it, and that's really hard to explain but I would absolutely know it. That would be my moment.
T: OK. So that would be…that's a big first signal.
C: Yeah.
T: What would the very first impact of that kind of realization be for you? How would that make a difference?
C: [Pause.] I guess the positive impact…normally when I go home I would take off everything before my ex-girlfriend would get home from work tonight, just because (a) she's not gonna be in my life anymore, (b) she's still a good person, I don't want her to question… don't wanna give her that confusion, like, I don't feel like I want to burden her with it.
T: Sure.
C: Umm, but I would actually just say, "I don't care," and just stay this way until she got home and have it not be a big deal.
T: OK.
C: I don't know. I think that would be a positive step, just go home and be like, well screw it, if she sees me like this, it's what it is. Without

having to feel like I need to explain it to her. But right now I feel like I would.

T: OK, so you would go home, and just stay you.

C: As is, absolutely.

T: OK.

C: Yeah, not really care what she thinks.

T: OK, anything before she gets home, that would be a further signal of this miracle? What else would be happening that would be significant, with this understanding and acceptance that you would have?

C: [Pause.] I can't...um I'm not too sure how to answer that without being redundant with what I've already said. I'm not really too sure how to elaborate.

T: So you're staying home, you're staying you? What would you do?

C: Play video games, have dinner, just be me 'cause that's my ultimate goal to just stay who I am as a person.

T: OK.

C: And keep my interests and everything like that, and just dress and be positive that I love heels and make-up and cute clothing. So yeah, I'd probably just continue as normal, just as I am right now [motioning to herself as a female], just as I'm dressed, as opposed to taking off everything.

T: So just be you, and do things that you already like doing, maybe play video games tonight.

C: Absolutely. That would be one of the best things. It doesn't need some big outer physical ceremony.

T: Yeah.

C: 'Cause that's not the goal; it's just to continue as I am, with the way that I want to look.

T: OK, so play video games. Any idea what you might play?

C: Mmm...probably Doda 2, it's basically a five versus five fantasy battle arena.

T: OK.

C: I'd probably play that, it's very competitive, very intense. It's a good one to use to kind of get lost in it. Which is how I use video games, it's just "Hey reality doesn't exist right now, I'm gonna play some video games."

T: Yeah. OK. So you would get lost in that.

C: Absolutely.

T: Any differences within that as a result of this miracle?

C: I'd probably change my profile name to be something more feminine. I'd probably just choose something else cuter than the one I have now.

T: OK.

C: That I would want to, and people on my friends list might be like "what? What is that?"

T: OK, changing your screen name?

C: Absolutely.

T: OK, anything else?

C: Probably post on Reddit's "ask transgender" about how good today felt. I don't know if you're aware…

T: I know Reddit, but not that topic.

C: It's just one of the sub Reddit's ask transgender it's just a community on there where it's just all discussion-based.

T: OK, so you would just post there.

C: Yeah, I'd post there about my experience, and maybe post a picture of how I look, 'cause many people want to see that 'cause it helps them with their struggles.

T: OK.

C: I would just post about the elation I was having and how good I felt about myself.

T: OK.

C: You're gonna tell me to go do all of this stuff aren't you?

T: I'm absolutely not.

C: [Laughs.]

T: [Laughing.] I'm just gonna keep asking questions.

C: [Still laughing.] OK.

T: Um. [Laughs.] So, OK, what would be the next signal, anything pre… um…what is your ex-girlfriend's name?

C: Christy.

T: Anything pre-Christy coming home, that would signify that this miracle has occurred within you?

C: Signals that I create, or signals that I notice? Either?

T: Yeah. That's a good distinction.

C: Well one, I was thinking, I would go to where I bought the wig from, and I'd buy the head mask for it, because I've been just keeping it in the bag it came in in the closet, which isn't good for it.

T: OK.

C: And I'd probably just have that up in the closet instead.

T: OK.

C: So that would be one I would create.

T: OK, OK so you would go and get that?

C: Yeah, just get the plastic head for it to sit on.

T: Yeah. OK, so just taking care of…

C: The hair.

T: Just that kind of thing?

C: Yeah and I might also like not hide my heels away in the closet either, just put them with my other shoes.

T: OK. So just being "out"?

C: Yeah. Absolutely.

T: OK.

C: Which I plan to do after she (Christy) leaves.

T: Yeah.

C: You know, when I move and I'm on my own. My plan is to like, you know work is like, boy-mode, because I'm only gonna be there for a year before I move, like, at least at this point in my life, I don't feel like I would need to go through the whole HR concerns, because of what that would mean.

T: Sure.

C: Um, and the other time I plan to go…so basically if you think of work and outside of work as 60/40, that's 60 percent of the time that I plan to go full-time, like this.

T: OK.

C: Except for work.

T: OK, so today you would start that 60 percent?

C: Absolutely, so it's the weekend, and I don't start work until the ninth, so I'd just be full time, I'd wake up and do my make-up everyday and if I was going to hang out with friends who are accepting of it… which I've done…only once but that was a fun experience, they were all very nice about it.

T: OK, so 60/40.

C: Yeah I would start that 60 percent today.

T: OK so shoes out, wig taken care of appropriately. Anything else that you would be taking care of that way?

C: I would have my make-up in the bathroom as opposed to stuffed away in a backpack.

T: OK. What difference would that make for you, to be able to be out at home?

C: It would feel really good.

T: Mm hmm.

C: I guess having those visual cues out in the open would help to reinforce the nature of what's going on here, rather than when you're pulling them out of somewhere. Like literally in the closet 'cause that's where I'm getting my wig.

T: Mm hmm.

C: Umm…[Laughing.] That's really funny, uhh…I didn't realize that. So yeah, it would help kind of reinforce it. Even if I'm not overtly thinking it as I see my make-up out on the counter, and stuff like that, it's just like subliminal, subconscious messages that you just see, where it's just 'normal'. It's not something I'm trying to hide.

T: The acceptance would just be there.

C: It would just be there, absolutely.

T: OK, um…alright, who do you think would be the first person who would notice this elation, this acceptance, who do you think would be the first person to notice this shift in you?

C: Probably Mark.

T: OK.

C: I don't see him in person, obviously, California, but we go on just computer voice chat programs. That's how we have kept being best friends since like 2000 I guess, and we're still best friends to this day. As if nothing's ever changed, really. I bet he would be able to notice it, even over voice chat.

T: Yeah? What would he notice, do you think?

C: I don't know, maybe just the tone in my voice. He would probably notice that I'm talking in a higher pitch. As opposed to talking [lowers voice to natural masculine tone] in my normal voice. Which I figured I could practice today 'cause it's non-judgmental.

T: Yeah, Yeah.

C: And I need practice, 'cause it's really fuckin' hard to maintain. [Laughing.]

T: Yeah.

C: But yeah, I think he would notice, maybe that, I mean that's just a sound cue, absolutely, but possibly just, I don't know, you know how when you're talkin' to someone over the phone and you can hear them smiling?

T: Mm hmm.

C: He would maybe even notice that, I believe, he's pretty perceptive on that.

T: OK. How would he let you know he saw this in you?

C: He'd probably just tell me. Like "hey man, you sound good. What's goin' on? You sound happy."

T: Nice. Alright. Who do you think would be the next person to notice this shift in you?

C: Nathan, but we don't hang out too often. He's super-busy.

T: OK.

C: But the next time we hung out he would notice, because if I were in this scenario, I'd be in my 60 percent.

T: What would Nathan notice, being physically present with you, other than the obvious appearance shift?

C: Probably just general attitude.

T: How do you mean?

C: Just a positivity I guess. Because before it was like, I came out to him, but I did it in boy-voice and boy-mode.

T: Yeah.

C: So I guess it would just be, "well this is where I'm at, I'm feeling good," I think he would be able to pick up on, just the positivity, I mean I don't want to sound all hippie, but surrounding me or something. [Laughing.]

T: OK, that makes sense. Like your aura?

C: Yeah, if you wanna use that word. [Laughing.] I was steering away from it but that's what I was thinking.

T: [Laughing.] OK so what other differences would you notice just in day-to-day life, you mentioned like when Christy comes home tonight, what would you notice about that. How would this miracle make a difference with her coming home?

C: [Pause.] I guess in my ability to explain it, it would be positive accepting and out, I guess I could say. It would just be another form of me being able to explain it and express it rather than just a frank conversation about it. If that makes sense.

T: OK, so it would be a positive and accepting and just matter of fact.

C: Yeah, and I believe it would be that anyway, but if I had this elation, oh I don't know, we keep going on with this scenario, and I'm gonna be there anyway, but putting it in right now, it would just be an easier way of explaining it to her, that's what the difference would be.

T: OK, you would be able to explain it more easily?

C: Yes, and comfortably, instead of just in short curt sentences. I'd be able to elaborate on it more.

T: OK, outside of Christy what would be the next signal to you. Tonight, or tomorrow, maybe going to sleep or waking up, that this miracle has occurred?

C: Well I don't think this would happen, but every morning when I wake up there's a few seconds between unconsciousness and consciousness where I wake up and I feel un-anxious before, well, I'm awake, and [snaps fingers] it's just like anxiety just kicks in, every morning no matter what.

T: OK.

C: So it's really complicated, so I don't think that I would be able to wake up and not have that feeling that I've been having for the last ten years, just the anxiety mode just kicks in and I have to control it once I wake up just to get back to a more leveled state.

T: OK.

C: But I don't know, theoretically what if that didn't happen? I just wake up and feel as calm as a person without a general anxiety disorder. Sure maybe you're like "oh something about the day might feel stressed out" but it's just like a physical weight that's on your chest that that just triggers a few moments after I wake up. It's very strange.

T: Mm hmm, so maybe you would wake up calm.

C: Yeah maybe I would wake up in that moment before that weight [snaps] falls, and it just doesn't, maybe it just hangs there and doesn't even come into contact with me. Even if it just hangs there for another 50 seconds as opposed to the first 10 seconds, even if it came after a minute.

T: OK.

C: Even if it just stayed off for a little bit more, before it fell. I think that would be a very positive notion that I didn't create because that's just something that happens.

T: OK. What difference would that make, to be able to wake up calm and stay calm?

C: Fucking, glorious. [Laughs.]

T: [Laughing.]

C: Um, it would feel like a new life, in a sense, even if it just stayed off for a little bit, before it clicked, that would just be a world of difference, that would let me know that this just gets easier, if I can go on and become more understanding with my own life, not even just in regard to transgender, just my life, that's just my life in general, that would make a world of a difference.

T: How would you notice that difference playing itself out?

C: Probably just that 50 seconds before the weight fell.

T: OK, what would you do with that?

C: Revel in it, maybe cry.

T: OK.

C: Or laugh.

T: If it stayed away?

C: Shhhh…[Shaking head and smiling.] [Whispers.] Oh God…

T: [Softly.] If this was the day when it stayed away?

C: I can't even imagine that…

T: Yeah.

C: Go ahead with your question, I'm just saying, I don't…I can't even picture it.

T: Umm…if you had to guess…if it stayed away…if you had to guess, like what would the next signal be after it stayed away…what would be the next signal that this was you, calm?

C: I guess a signal that I created next would be that I would just get rid of the cigarettes in my car, instead of just leaving them there as a precautionary measure. Just being like, I really don't need this…that would be the next big trigger I guess, that would set in motion that this was gone, the anxiety.

T: OK, so the cigarettes would be gone?

C: Yeah, they would be absolutely gone; I would have no desire for them.

T: OK. What else would be different about calm, April?

C: That's hard to even picture.

T: Sure. If you had to guess?

C: [Pause and sigh.] Hopefully not thinking that every single little pain in my body would lead to a full-blown anxiety attack. I guess that calm would hopefully help to quell the hypochondria.

T: OK. So if you got a pain somewhere…

C: It would just be "welp…that's just a pain, whatever, my arm fell asleep randomly, it's not that I'm having a heart attack."

T: OK, so you'd just kind of shake it off?

C: Yeah it would be no big deal.

T: OK.

C: So yeah, that would be the next involuntary trigger, because it would have to happen to where I wouldn't consciously try to calm myself down after feeling something, it would just have to happen, with me realizing it after the fact.

T: So just being able to be OK with random pain happening, and moving on?

C: Yeah, 'cause I'm definitely not opposed to pain, I've got tattoos, and like I even went and got my underarms waxed, I'm not opposed to physical pain.

T: But it would be very different for you, to experience a random pain, and just be fine with it, and move on?

C: Yeah, I wouldn't have to recite my name out loud to make sure I wasn't having a stroke.

T: OK, so your mind would be 'here.'

C: Absolutely.

T: OK. Any other signals of calm?

C: Those are the major ones.

T: OK. Anything else about this miracle comfort, elation, acceptance, anything else about this version of you kind of at your best, that you want to touch on that you think you would notice?

C: No, those are the major points.

T: OK.

The importance of tenacity

As you can see within this transcript, clients might have a hard time envisioning the smaller details of their miracle day, and it is up to the practitioner to gently keep probing until they get the information they are seeking. As I was asking April about this day, and was seeking smaller details between the time when she got home and when her ex-girlfriend got home, she started off a bit confused, and thus not really answering my question. So I clarified a bit by breaking it down further and asking what she would be doing specifically, and within those details she was quite easily able to talk about what differences she would notice, and those differences became pretty significant. From changing her video game persona, to sharing her elation with others online, to taking better care of her clothes, make-up, wig, and shoes. These significant details may not have emerged if I had given up when she first said she didn't know what she would notice.

And later, when April was talking about waking up calm, and staying calm, if this miracle resulted in a day when that anxiety never – as she put it – dropped, she had a very hard time imagining that as a possibility. So

I simply asked her to guess what it might be like, and she was able to then elaborate about this calm version of herself, who stays present-focused throughout her day. As a therapist seeking these details it is very important to practice this sort of tenacity, sticking with a question once you know it's a good one until the client comes up with a description you can build on.

Clients may continue answering in problem-language for a while, or simply say that they aren't sure and sit quietly until the clinician asks something else. I think one of the most common mistakes with newer SF clinicians is that they allow their client's initial uncertainty to cause them to abandon the question they are asking altogether, and maybe even follow the client into problem-land rather than sticking to the question and tenaciously seeking detail after detail. Without complete trust in this question – and thus tenacity as you seek the answers – building solutions can become a very difficult task.

Conclusion

The miracle question and the subsequent details that follow are the heart of the initial solution-focused conversation. And with the LGBT community, the tenacity and discipline with which a clinician asks the miracle question and elicits detail after detail of their client's preferred future as they hope it to be, is key to helping that client move forward in a way that is right for them. From best hopes, to connecting, to this preferred future description, the client has been in the driver's seat the whole way, with the therapist using discipline, tenacity, and respectful curiosity throughout. By the time you finish getting the details of the preferred future, you're very close to the finish line of the first session. But as you're about to see, the work is not quite done yet.

6   Scaling

The best thing about the future is that it comes one day at a time.
(Abraham Lincoln, Students' Academy, 2014)

Typically with about 10–15 minutes left in the session, you've got a good detailed picture of the client's miracle day, and it's time to find out what's already happening in your client's life that they are happy with, and then discuss how they might notice the next small steps forward. In SFBT we do both of these things with one useful little tool: the scale.

The scale is perfect for measuring all kinds of life situations and hopes that your client comes into therapy with. "They can be used to access the client's perception of almost anything" (De Jong and Berg, 2008, p. 107). And with the LGBT community there are a lot of very unique opportunities to use scales. I'll get into those later in the chapter, but first I'll explain a bit about how scales are used in SFBT, and the miracle scale.

Solution-focused scaling

Scales are certainly not unique to SFBT. Many practitioners use scaling as a tool for measuring where their client is in relation to a problem, or the pain they are experiencing. However, scaling in SFBT is a bit different than scaling in a more problem-focused session, because an SF scale is not in relation to a problem; rather it is in relation to our clients' preferred future. In SFBT the scale goes from zero to ten, where zero equals nothing about the miracle picture is happening at all, and ten represents the day the client has just described to you happening in totality.

The miracle scale

Identifying current placement on the scale

Asking an initial scaling question in regards to the miracle is quite simple, but it has a couple of very important components involved that will help the client to answer more precisely. The first thing to do is define the scale for the client. You do that by saying something a bit like this:

> OK, so think about a scale of zero to ten, where ten equals everything that we've just talked about in your miracle day is happening as you've just described, and zero is the exact opposite. Where would you say you are right now on that scale?

Notice that the ten is defined quite clearly in that question, yet zero is only defined as "the exact opposite." This is simply because it isn't necessary or particularly helpful to give any more details about what zero means. We do this very much on purpose, as a means of continuing the flow of the solution-building process without getting off-track into problem-talk.

Also, in the question as it is posed above, you see "right now" as the reference point for where the client is. With many clients within the LGBT community, I've noticed that when I specify, "right now," as opposed to something more general like "today," they think for a minute and give an answer that they sometimes say was lower just before coming into the session. I had a client who identified as a trans-male tell me that when he came in he would have said he was at a two, but after having detailed a day where he was confident and comfortable just being himself, moving towards transition and building the life he always wanted, he already felt more confident and able to do some of what he had just described moving forward, and he realized through our conversation that he was closer now than he had initially realized to making that preferred future become a reality. So he said at that exact moment he would put himself at a five. If I had said "today," or even asked him where he thought he had been over the last few days, he probably would have given me a lower number – and that incredible three-point swing up, and recognition of the shifts that have already happened, might have been missed.

In *More than Miracles*, the authors point out that "The scale also transforms the miracle from an endpoint to a series of steps – a process whereby each step contains thoughts, emotions, behaviors, and interactions in different areas of the client's life and reality" (de Shazer et al., 2007, p. 61). This distinction between an endpoint and a series of steps is incredibly important when the client is at the beginning of what can necessarily be a several-year process, such as gender transition. Often, when transgender clients think of their "ten," they picture themselves fully transitioned and thus able to be their true selves 100 percent of the time. And that can understandably feel very far away and quite daunting. But scaling in this way can help that client break down transition into these smaller and more manageable stages, where everything is affected positively as forward movement takes place.

April's miracle scale, step one

T: OK April, so, on a scale of zero to ten, where ten is this accepting, elated, comfortable, confident version of you, and zero is the exact opposite. Where would you say you are on the scale right now?
C: Right now?
T: Yeah.
C: [Pause.] Six or seven.
T: OK.
C: I would say, like I feel really good about where I'm at, but I know I could make progress in that area. But I'm definitely not on the bottom side of five in that regard.

You'll notice that when I defined "ten," I went back to April's specified best hopes from our work together. I did not define ten as "fully transitioned" or using any other language. It is very important to stay with the client's very best hopes with the miracle scale, and let them be the ones who define what that will look like practically.

Using scales to elicit exceptions

Once you have the current placement on the scale, the very next question you ask can feel a little bit counterintuitive for anyone who's only ever used scales in a problem-focused way. April's transcript is a good example of what I mean:

T: So you feel really good. What else signifies to you that you're as high as a six or a seven, instead of on the bottom side of five?
C: That I'm here.
T: OK. [Pause, purposefully, to elicit more information.]
C: That I'm dressed. [Motioning to herself dressed as a female.] I'd say those are my biggest signals, that I can just discuss this without having some sort of a panic attack. Or just that I don't' think it's really a trigger at all. I don't have any anxiety per se.
T: OK, so you're here, and you can talk about it openly?
C: Yeah, absolutely.
T: OK, any other signals that you're as high as a six or seven already?
C: No, I just feel good about how I look.
T: OK.
C: I guess that, yeah, would be a point, that I feel confident.
T: OK.
C: But I know I can go higher.

Notice how I used the *exact* words she did when initially asking her this question; she segued perfectly into this question when she said she knew she wasn't on the "bottom side of five," and I picked up those exact words to seek a descriptor of what she is *already* doing well. Even when a client answers with a lower number than April did – maybe saying they are at a two or a one – the next question should always be, "How do you know you're as high as a two, rather than a one or zero?" This question elicits things that are already going well in your client's life, things they may not even be fully conscious of but that are very important to note.

When the client says "zero"

Sometimes clients come in incredibly distressed, and they might say that they feel like they are at a zero or even a negative number on that scale. I had a client once who was going through an incredibly tough break-up and subsequent depression so that she thought she was at a minus 26 on a scale of zero to ten. Here are some tips for addressing these types of answers:

- Address the difficulty the client is clearly articulating to you, by saying something along the lines of, "Wow, it seems like things are very tough at the moment."
- Ask something along the lines of, "How are you stopping things from getting worse?"
- Ask what is helping them to get through this tough time. My client who said "minus 26" said that her dog was what helped her the most. Having her dog, who loved her and who she loved back, to care for on a daily basis was what helped her get through the day.
- Scale safety. I asked my client about safety, feeling very concerned about her current situation. I asked her on a scale of zero to ten – where ten was that although things were difficult, she was completely able to keep herself safe, and zero was the opposite, that she was suicidal and didn't think she could keep herself safe. She said she was at an eight, she knew this was going to take some time but that eventually she would get through it, and she wanted to keep moving so that she could see the other side of this terrible place she was in. If a client says they are unable to keep themselves safe, it might be a good idea to put therapy aside for a bit, and determine the right course of action from there to help ensure the client doesn't act on their suicidality.
- Move on to the next small signs of progress as outlined below.

Pre-session change

Sometimes, either at this point in the session or even closer to the start of it, clients will mention some changes that have already begun, before the session even got started. I was talking with a family for the first time recently, and mom and dad had been incredibly worried about their son. And when it was time to scale where things were at the moment, their son said he was at a four. His mom chimed in at that point – before I could ask my next question – and asked where he thought he had been the week before, and he said a one. His parents nodded in agreement, and his dad specified that they thought just getting their son an appointment scheduled, so that he could finally talk to someone, seemed to help him feel more hopeful the minute they told him they'd scheduled.

This often happens with couples as well – just the act of scheduling what they assume will be a helpful therapy session with a counselor sometimes begins to create the change in their relationship they were hoping to create through the therapy. Highlighting this progress with questions can not only serve to point out the progress itself, but help clients to recognize that they are already moving towards their preferred future, before even talking with the person they've hired to help them do just that.

You can elicit this information in a few different ways, such as:

- "What have you noticed, just since the call you made to schedule, that you've been pleased with?"
- "Where would you say you were on the scale before calling? [and once they answer] And what about after calling but just before coming in?"

Next small steps

OK, so you've got an answer to where the client is right now on their scale, and you know what they feel happy with and how they know they are as high as they are. The next task an SF practitioner has is to have the client identify the next small steps towards that miracle picture they've just described. You do this by asking about how the client would notice moving forward just one number higher on the scale, no more than that. This tiny movement helps the client to think very small, and therefore give details of some small, quite achievable steps that they might take in the coming days.

In the session with April, she had a *very* hard time thinking about the next small steps forward. Between the question and her eventual answer, we sat in *complete* silence for a full minute, while she considered her answer. I have to admit that I was a bit nervous in that silence, hoping against hope that she would finally think of some small step. But when she spoke, she came up with some signals that were quite meaningful to her, and I was so very glad that I had been patient and allowed myself to feel that discomfort, rather than saying anything to break her train of thought or just outright deciding to believe her when she initially said she couldn't answer the question.

April's transcript, the next small step

T: OK, you just led me to my next question. If that six or seven turned into a seven or eight, so that you spend a few days at a seven or an eight, how would you notice just a little bit better? Not a nine or ten, just a little bit better, how would you notice?

C: I can't really answer that right now, I'm not really sure. I would have to notice it, to be able to notice it, I'm not sure if I can just theorize right now, what it would be.

T: Any small guesses? [Pause.] Some little tiny movement forward for you? Signals of that?

C: [Pause for 15 seconds.] I'm still not sure how to answer you.

T: Keep thinking; take as much time as you need. [Pause.] You don't have to be right; you just have to guess, like how would you...

C: Yeah absolutely.

T: What might be happening to let you know, that the six or seven is definitely a solid seven or maybe a seven and a half, just a little bit closer to your best-self.

C: [Pause for a full 60 seconds while the therapist silently sweats in her seat and remains very still.]...I don't know I guess maybe in terms of practical application it would be feeling comfortable enough to go and actually get a...I know it sounds silly but...a better manicure, as a boy, but being comfortable to wear it in both 60 and my 40. To where it's nothing crazy, maybe it's a nice cream white French, but not being like, "ah they're just going to judge me because I have a French manicure as a boy" and just being OK with that, as long as it doesn't' affect me like, getting fired or something like that.

T: OK.

C: 'Cause if it's not like a big deal at work I would absolutely do that, just have it, 'cause I would love to have nicer nails. I went and got a manicure but they just buffed it to make it shinier, I would love to have like a coat, on there.

T: OK.

C: I don't know if that...

T: Yeah, no that is exactly the kind of thing.

C: OK.

T: That's perfect, OK.

C: I guess that would help me like graduate from that, 'cause it's another step towards not just a 60/40 but an eventual 100.

T: OK.

C: Which I guess, to put this on an actual timeline, it would be like California, like California would be like the actual 100 – one, because of their laws about hiring, and two, hopefully by that time I would already be like on five months of a low dose of HRT or something, and, um, it's just a timeline picture I have.

T: OK, so any steps that you would make towards that 100…
C: Absolutely.
T: Would be signals to you.
C: Yeah, so it's just the nails, 'cause the nails would then become 100, so that's just one further step towards 100. Like another step that I've taken, which is why I'm at a six or seven, is being confident enough to wear jewelry in boy mode, it doesn't matter if I got it in the woman's section, it's just wearing it even without the make-up and the wig, and being absolutely comfortable with that.

April was able to identify a small step, getting a French manicure, and the feelings she would associate with that step: comfort and confidence. As the therapist, the most important piece of that information is not the step itself, but the positive feelings the client imagines that step will create. Whatever it is that creates those feelings will be significant for April, a point we will explore a bit further in Chapter 7.

Other solution-focused scales

One of the things I love most about these scales is how they reinforce the client as the expert and keep them in control of defining where they are and where they hope to be. In sessions with every type of client, but especially with the LGBT community, there are many different uses for scaling throughout SF sessions.

I was recently working with a 16-year-old kid who felt like they might truly identify as transgender, but both they and their parents were very uncertain if that was really what was going on with them. This kid's parents were completely terrified for their child, and what this possible identity would mean for them as an adolescent in a small Texas town. When the kid came in to talk with me, they said their hope was to get some clarity so that they could figure themselves out, and then gain the confidence to move towards transition if in fact they really were transgender. During one of our sessions, with the parents and teen in the room, I asked the teenager to scale their certainty about being transgender, where ten was they were 100 percent sure they identified as transgender and zero was they were not sure at all. They thought about it for a minute and finally answered with the number four. I heard the mother sigh with relief, and I looked over at her, and tearing up a bit she said that she was so happy to hear the number four because it meant they all had a little more time. I asked what she meant and she said one of the most loving things I've ever heard a parent say. She said that if her kid, who she had always assumed was a girl, turned out to truly be a boy, a son, she wanted to help him to do whatever needed doing to feel comfortable in his own body, and to be happy and successful in life, whether that meant beginning hormones, changing his name to match his identity, coming out at school, whatever he wanted or needed. She said she was ready as soon as her kid told her they were ready, but hearing the number four took a bit of the pressure off and let her know they still had time to figure out the next steps as a family, and get used to the idea of what those steps might mean.

I looked over at the teenager sitting in the opposite chair, and saw tears streaming down their face. They said that hearing their mother say those things let them know that whatever it was that was happening with them, they were going to be OK because mom would be there to help. One of their biggest fears was that their family wouldn't be supportive, if in fact they did come out as transgender. When I saw that family again a few months later the teen had come out as a transgender male to his family, and the first thing he said when I saw him was that he was sure about who he was and his certainty was now at a nine. He said that knowing his mother had his back made all the difference in the world for him to truly be honest about what he was going through and he was able to explore his masculinity more fully at home by doing things like asking his parents to call him his preferred name as well as male gender pronouns, and other little things like not shaving his legs or underarms, all of which increased his confidence and thus his certainty that this truly was the right path for him.

Any time you have a client who is unsure about their gender or sexuality, scaling can be an incredibly useful tool for helping them to clarify, both to themselves and sometimes even their loved ones, just how sure they are, and then any forward movement they make at all is clearer as a result, and can be built on over time.

Other LGBT scales

Extent of transition

This scale can be useful when a transgender client is hoping to recognize progress and stay motivated even throughout the sometimes very slow transition towards their true self. Many times the next small step might not move them from a 4 to a 5, but from a 4 to a 4.1, and just realizing that tiny movement can sometimes help folks to realize they really are making progress. Further, this scale is important because ten is always defined by the client, so it will always be different for each client who uses it. Ten might mean fully transitioned, with medications and surgery to one client; but to another it might mean just HRT and a legal name change.

Readiness to come out

Many LGBT clients feel pressured to come out at work or to loved ones, before they are ready. Sometimes I'll scale their readiness with them to get an idea of where they are on that scale, which keeps them in control, with questions like, "What number would you like to be at before you start to make moves towards coming out?"

Readiness to transition

Every client is different, and sometimes they want to transition sooner in the process than others, and other clients might want to (or need to for financial or legal reasons) wait a bit longer.

Masculinity or femininity

Gender is *much* more complicated than zero to ten; however, sometimes a scale as black and white as that one is useful for clients who are trying to discover who they really are in their gender or gender expression. With this scale, zero can be as masculine as one can be, and ten as feminine as one can be, or vice versa.

Sexuality

Similar to gender, sexuality is also more complicated than a zero to ten, but sometimes a scale can help clients to see where they might really be, and how they might identify if they are feeling unclear. With sexuality, zero might be as straight as one can be and ten as gay, with five being bisexual or pansexual.

Relationship with loved ones (where ten is the relationship they want to have)

Many clients talk about wanting a closer relationship with their family or friends, or even their partner, once they've come out or begun to transition. I was recently talking with a woman who just came out as lesbian to her parents, and she realized that her mother was very distant in a way she had never been before. She was talking about how this difference was troubling to her, so I asked her to scale where she thought the relationship was, if ten was the relationship she wanted to have with her mother, given the reality of the difficult situation they were in. She thought for a moment, and then she said, "Actually, I'd say our relationship is an eight, I know my mom well, and I know she's going to need a little more time before we're back to talking every day, but I'm OK enough with where it is now." She was surprised to hear herself say that, but putting it on the scale helped her realize its truth.

Readiness to begin dating

Clients who have just come out, or just got out of a tough relationship, are sometimes feeling pressure to begin dating either by peers or well-meaning family members, but just aren't sure if they're ready. This is a useful scale to clarify just how ready they are.

Conclusion

As you can see, scales can be used in many situations with LGBT clients. Clarity scales such as gender or sexuality or hope scales, where ten will always equal the hope being realized, and zero the opposite. Every single one of these scales is used to keep the client in the driver's seat, and can continue to be addressed throughout the course of therapy, so that clients can keep clarifying and even identify the next small steps forward for each hope they express.

7 Feedback, homework, and closing the initial session

Success is achieved by development of our strengths, not by elimination of our weaknesses.

(Marilyn Vos Savant, 2014)

At this point, there are typically only a few minutes left in the session, and it's time to start conceptualizing what you've learned about this client throughout the last hour. Sometimes SF clinicians will take a brief break here to get their thoughts together and really think about what they've just learned about this individual, couple, or family. They might take a minute to think on what evidence have they gathered that lets them know this client is totally capable of moving towards the preferred future they've just described, asking themselves a question such as, "What are this client's strengths, values, resources, and talents?"

Looking back at April's transcript, think about what you have learned about her. If you took a second to write down what has impressed you about her, based solely on her answers to the questions throughout the transcript, I imagine you could come up with some pretty important values she clearly holds dear, and some unique strengths and talents she's seemingly used quite effectively thus far in her life. She has overcome depression, she's on the path to overcoming some pretty serious anxiety, she's currently coping quite well with the loss of a job and a meaningful relationship just in the past few months, not to mention this new "horizon" as she's put it, that she's beginning to walk towards, that could mean turning her world on its head. Her strength, intelligence, and self-awareness are clear attributes she's used to navigate quite successfully through this incredibly tumultuous time in her life.

Here is what I noticed about April, and the feedback I gave her as a result:

April's transcript: feedback

T: So, you're very impressive to me, April, and I'd like to tell you why, if it's OK.

C: Sure, that sounds great, I love being called impressive. [Laughing.]

T: [Laughing.] And after that I want to, um…

C: The bad?

T: No, no, absolutely not bad things, I just want to ask you to be on the lookout for some things.

C: Oh, sure.

T: Um…so…it's clear to me that you, or that analytical side of you, it seems as if you've found a way to turn the analytical side, the side that used to cause some issues for you, to turn it into a strength. It seems like you've taken the analytical and turned it into, glass half-full thinking. You've made a conscious choice to analyze in a way that is helpful to you, in a way that is productive for you, in a way that gets you through work, and in a way that helps you get through struggles at home, and in a way that helps you with every-day mundane things, but also very much in a way that helps you to become your true self. So you haven't changed yourself, you've taken this thing about you, you know yourself very well, and you've taken this thing about you and you've molded it.

C: And I got there because of the analytical thinking. That's the only way that I could get there.

T: Yeah, and it's just very impressive, it's clear to me that you've turned this into your absolute biggest strength, and it is a huge strength to wield, it seems. It seems like this is an absolutely huge strength for you, I mean you are seemingly at a point of acceptance in all of this, having just, you said, realized this in the last couple of months…

C: One.

T: …The last month, the last couple of weeks then, to be able to go from coming out to yourself, to being able to come as far as you have in the last month.

C: That just means it's always been there, it's just been ready.

T: Yeah.

C: It's been locked and loaded.

T: Yeah, um, it seems as though you are just kind of coming into yourself, quite literally, actually, but also emotionally and psychologically, and it seems clear to me just based on the conversation we just had, and it's just very impressive. Um, so it also seem like you're doing some things that are very, very good for you, you're making some decisions that are very good for you, even if they are not the easiest decisions, like waiting to tell mom and dad. You very specifically have an idea of "this is what I need to do, because I know my mom well enough to know that this is going to be best, for me and for our relationship. So I'm gonna wait, though it may not be easy, and then do it the right way." And do it in a way that is very, very, very caring of yourself. You are clearly very confident, and you know yourself well enough to know what is good for you, and what is not good for you, and you are willing to do things the right way so that you are OK, and just kind of caring for yourself in those ways. I mean you've come a really, really long way, from, when you had a little bit of depression and anxiety that you've had in the past, you've conquered a whole lot, just to get this far in your life, and it seems as though that is all…

C: I've never taken medication either.

T: Yeah? Wow, it seems like all of that has just snowballed into this ability that you have to come as far as you have in a matter of weeks. You're somebody who, when you know what you want, it seems as though you just go, and you get it.

C: [Pointing at the therapist.] You're gonna tell me to not go too fast, I believe, right? Is that a thing to watch out for?

T: Nah.

C: OK.

T: That's up to you.

C: That's just me again being analytical, like "well you're saying I'm going fast, like well, hmm. I gotta make sure I don't go too fast though."

T: Well you're already kind of checkin' that with yourself though, you're already checkin' that.

C: I don't wanna lose myself in it, I just wanna mold the two together.

T: Yeah you're seemingly kind of doing that already within yourself, so I mean I don't have any specific advice for you as far as how to go about this, I think that you're going about it in an incredible way.

The purpose of feedback

In SFBT, feedback is never about being critical of the client. As you can see in the transcript, there was certainly an opportunity for me to advise April to go slowly, but it never even crossed my mind because that would have been taking away her credit. Effective solution-focused feedback, or compliments, are "not in the compliment itself but in the evidence to the client, expressed through the compliment, that the coach is listening in a very different way to that which was expected" (Iveson et al., 2012a, p. 108). April is already doing things to go at a pace that is right for her; she is checking herself regularly and doing a really good job of moving forward. Giving her advice about how to go about this would have completely negated everything she was already doing, and made the entire session feel like I had been analyzing her moves and being critical of them the entire time, rather than just listening with respectful curiosity. So rather than do that at all, I just wanted her to know what I learned about her ability to go about this in a way that was absolutely right for her, let her know that it's clear to me that she's already doing some things very well. At this point the 'therapy' per se has already been done, the conversation we had has just done all the work that there is to do, and all I'm trying to do is to let her know what I have learned about her, to drive home her strengths and skills, and then to get out of there without negating all of the work that has already happened.

A lesson in leading from behind

Something else I want to point out here is to never make any assumptions about where your client will end up on this journey they are on. With clients who come in uncertain about their gender identity or sexual orientation, it is incredibly important to keep respecting them as the experts over that often incredibly complex process. April is on a journey of discovering her gender identity. She came in dressed as her female self, and continues to refer to that version of herself as being in "girl-mode." Therefore I continually use female pronouns with her. But she made it quite clear when she came in that she hadn't yet fully discovered her true gender identity, and that she was not yet 100 percent sure that she fully identified as a transgender female. It is very important for counselors working with gender and sexual minorities who are still at a point of questioning their identity, to never go so far as to assume they know better than their clients, where that client will end up.

Sometimes a well-meaning therapist might think, "There's certainly nothing wrong with being gay or transgender, so fully accepting this client as that, even before they have accepted it themselves, must be the right thing to do." But that thinking immediately takes the client out of the driver's seat, and in the cases where that client ends up not identifying as gay or transgender, they might feel like they've disappointed you, and that in itself can create problems. Never get ahead of your clients, rather always lead from behind, with questions that simply build on what they've already said, and then you will never get to a place before they have, ensuring that you don't end up in the wrong place ahead of them, unable to meet them if they happen to swerve in an unexpected direction. In Chapter 8 I'll offer a follow-up with April that will highlight and explain this even further.

Homework

This brings us to the homework step, and again I definitely don't want to negate the work that's already been accomplished so I go about this very carefully and thoughtfully as well.

Here's April's transcript as an example of what I mean:

April's transcript: homework

T: The one thing that I would ask you to do, is to keep noticing your presence on this scale, notice anything that you do that lets you know that you're moving forward.
C: Even the smallest things?

T: Especially the smallest things.

C: OK, I will actually take notes, in my phone, and just have it there.

T: Yeah, so any signals to you that you are moving toward that understanding and confidence. Any signals that you're moving forward, and then the positive impacts that they have on you. So if you do get a manicure or anything like that, I imagine that might have some positive ripple effects throughout every tiny little piece of your day, pay attention to that stuff.

C: OK.

T: The very first question that I'm going to ask you, should you choose to come back here, is "What's been better since I saw you last," so that's why I want you to pay attention.

C: OK.

T: And we'll go from there.

C: OK.

T: Sound good?

C: That sounds fantastic.

The homework of 'noticing'

So that's it, no big homework assignment to do anything specific at all, we aren't setting goals here, we are just talking about noticing progress towards the client's preferred future in real time, as it happens, whatever it might be that creates it. This type of minimalist homework assignment in SFBT originated in London, with BRIEF, and in their book *Brief Coaching*, the authors point out that "It can be argued that what we notice as we go around our worlds is the inevitable basis for us to reach certain identity conclusion" (Iveson et al., 2012a, p. 106). Thus, noticing forward movement towards our preferred future can help us to reach that very future.

Remember back in the transcript where April and I were scaling where she was, and she asked me if I was going to tell her to leave and go and do those things? See here that I definitely did not do that. I did mention the manicure, when I said that if she does go to do that, to notice if that has positive ripple effects; but I did not tell her to go and get a manicure, nor would I ever tell a client to go and do anything specific like that. The reason I wouldn't is because until the client notices what she does that works, I simply cannot know what will. In April's case, for all I know what might end up helping her to increase her understanding and confidence has nothing at all to do with getting a manicure. And as a therapist who wants the client to stay firmly in the driver's seat from the word go, I don't want to pretend to know what might work. So, we simply ask them to notice forward movement, and we leave it at that, allowing them to choose what to do and notice what works on their own.

Let me use another example to amplify what I mean here.

Craig

I remember meeting Craig in the summer of 2011, as he was trying to get though a tough break-up. Throughout the first session, and as he was describing his preferred future, he kept referencing going to his old Alcoholics Anonymous meetings again, and socializing in healthy ways through them. So at the end of the session I asked him to notice what worked, to help him move forward in the coming week, and when I saw him at the next session he said things were a little better. I asked him to elaborate, and he said that he went to church for the first time in several years. He remembered after our first session that he didn't go to those AA meetings anymore because as much as he wanted them to be healthy for him, those actual meetings typically ended up not being healthy at all. So he went to church instead, and the positive social impacts he was looking for happened as a result. If I had told Craig to go to a meeting as his homework, it might have made it harder for him to find the right solution that following week – but staying out of the way completely allowed him to just focus on what might work, and do what he thought was best, and then to notice what worked.

The homework of trying an 'experiment'

When I work with individuals, couples, and families within the transgender community, the idea of 'experiments' comes up a lot in-session. When a client has just come out as transgender, and hasn't yet begun to medically transition with hormone replacement therapy, but believes that they want to, then beginning HRT is simply seen as an 'experiment' until the client can determine the impact HRT has after they take it. When I am talking with the parents of a transgender teen, we might try the experiment of using the teen's preferred pronouns around the house, or coming up with a more gender-appropriate name that the teen is comfortable with. Seeing these small steps as experiments leaves the door open for the individual to see the experiment as a failure, or as a success, depending on the impacts of the experiment – without feeling too attached to the step itself. However, it is important to remember that the desire to begin to transition socially or medically, must first come from the client when they are ready to move forward in that way.

Closing the session and scheduling another

The final utterances of the first session are about scheduling the next session, but again, there is something a little bit different about how this is done in an SF session, so I wanted to add it here.

April's transcript: following up

T: OK, I would love to follow up if you think it would be helpful.
C: OK.
T: So what do you want to do? [Grabbing phone for calendar.]
C: As far as coming back?
T: Yeah, it's totally up to you.
C: I'm not sure what would be helpful in terms of giving it enough time to move from the six or seven, I don't think a week would be enough, maybe three weeks or a month...
T: OK, it's totally up to you.
C: Um, lets go for a month.
T: OK.
C: And if something happens I can schedule for sooner, but we can just go for a month.
T: OK.

This is another tip I once got from Elliott that stuck with me. It is my belief that wherever possible, and certainly in private practice, clients should always dictate when and how often they come in for therapy. I give April 100 percent control over scheduling the next appointment – I don't suggest anything at all, except that I'd love to follow up if she thinks it would be helpful. I do this for every single client that I see, and while it may not always be the smartest financial decision to leave this up to my clients, it is certainly the most in-line way of scheduling subsequent session within solution-focused practice. Sometimes clients will say, "I'll get back to you about rescheduling," or even, "I'm feeling really good, I don't know if I need another appointment," and whether it's because the session has been very helpful, or not helpful at all, the best way I've found to make space for the client to remain in the driver's seat is to always leave it open in this way.

Conclusion

By this point in the session most of the work has been completed, and the best thing to do is reinforce the work you and the client have already done and get out of the session without negating any of it.

8   Subsequent sessions

Don't judge each day by the harvest you reap, but by the seeds you plant.
(Robert L. Stevenson, Students' Academy, 2015)

So, you've had one session with your LGBT client, and sometime later they come back, ready to continue. In many trainings on solution-focused therapy there is very little about what to do after session number one. There are so many important pieces to cover about SFBT in general, and the first session itself, that by the time you get to the subsequent sessions there is typically little to no time left to talk about them in depth, and how to keep your questions in line with those assumptions, tenets, and principles as clients' lives shift from one dynamic to another, throughout the course of therapy. But the reality is that with many clients the time you spend with them will be much more than just the first hour, and I think clinicians are done a disservice when they aren't taught more in depth about how to carry solution-building conversations forward from the second session through to the last. I believe it is important because of how challenging it can be to continue the solution-focused conversations session after session.

I recently had a client come in as an individual after trying months of couples' counseling with another therapist – a person that my client described as an older man and an old school therapist. She said that after a few sessions he recommended that she find a female counselor to help her get through the trust issues she was continuing to have with her husband of 25 years. She came in to see me and one of the first things she asked was for me to explain SFBT to her. She said that when she told her therapist about setting up an appointment with me, and described to him what my website said about my therapy style, he said, "She must be very smart. That is a very hard therapy style to do." I'm not sure exactly what that therapist meant, but I do have a guess. I think it might have to do with two specific things; one is that the longer into your career it is when you try to learn SFBT, the more you will have to *unlearn* in order to be able to do SFBT effectively. And for a therapist who has been practicing for 20 years or more and who was described as "very old school," it would make complete sense for him to see that as quite a challenge. Also, I would guess that he might have meant that sticking purely to SFBT session after session requires a *lot* of discipline and quite a bit of skill, and I would agree with that wholeheartedly. However, sticking to the assumptions and tenets when a client has come back to you time and time again is just as important as sticking to them in that first session.

Throughout this chapter are some client stories and transcripts to outline each piece of a follow-up session. And then at the end of the chapter I'll provide an update on what happened in the three follow-up sessions I had with April.

Signs of progress

Subsequent sessions in SFBT, whether it's session 2 or 25, all start with some version of this question: "What's been better, even just a little bit, since we last spoke?" The clear assumption behind this question is that somehow, something must have worked effectively in the days since the client has seen you, and the purpose behind asking it is to keep the solution-building conversation from the previous session moving forward.

Often the individual, couple, or family is able to easily answer this question with things that they've noticed since the last meeting. If you remember in the transcript from Chapter 7, I warned April that I would ask this question, very purposefully setting her up to notice the progress she made; and often this warning helps clients to be ready for the question when it's asked in follow-ups, and thus have an answer ready. Sometimes, though, the client might say that nothing has been better, or, in fact, that things have been worse since the last session. In this case, the respectful tenacity I've touched on throughout this book is incredibly important, and a bit of creativity can help here.

Let me outline this with two case examples; one of a lesbian couple I worked with a couple of years ago, and the next with an individual gay male I worked with throughout last year.

Natasha and Latoya

I first met with Natasha and Latoya in the winter of 2012. They came in hoping to get back to the loving couple they had once been, where they were affectionate, patient, and open with each other. In our first conversation they each detailed a picture of their preferred future where they were prioritizing each other again, going out on dates like they used to, and finding intimacy desirable. When we met for our second session a week later, I asked them what had been better since our first session. With folded arms, and sitting on the opposite side of the couch from each other, they both said firmly that nothing was better, and in fact things were much worse as a result of a fight they'd had the day before our session. I responded by noting that it seemed very clear that things were feeling pretty tough for the couple at the moment, and then followed up with, "But can you think of any instance in the last week, where things were better, even just a little bit?" And again, the response came hard and cold from each of them that "no, we cannot think of a single instance of better." So I thought for a second, and then stood up and walked over to a whiteboard I had hanging up on my wall, and I drew a little graph with the weekdays between our last session and that one along the bottom from left to right; and the numbers zero to ten going along the left side with "10" on top and "0" on the bottom. I then asked them to recall the number they said they were at during our last session, and they agreed they were at a four last time. I put a little dot that corresponded to that first Saturday on the graph, and the number four. I asked them what they would say Sunday was, on that same zero to ten, and they agreed that it stayed at a four. I went on to Monday, and they said it went down to a three then, and stayed at a three throughout the week until Thursday night. When I got to Thursday, I asked where it was and they both said it was at a seven from Thursday until late that Friday evening, when it dropped to a two due to a fight. At that point I looked at the graph and had a whole lot of possibilities for questions swimming through my mind – so I decided to start on that first Saturday, and asked them how they knew it stayed at a four from Saturday to Sunday, before dropping down to that three. They said they went to lunch after our session, had a good talk about their future, and both of them recommitted to really trying to work things out. They decided that day that they would give this a real shot at working, and that commitment from both of them was helpful. They said that Latoya spent the night with Natasha that night, something she hadn't done in weeks, and they got along well throughout the evening and on Sunday, when Natasha made them brunch at home and they ate and talked about plans for their future. Then, Latoya said something pretty remarkable: "You know, now that I think about it, I'd give Sunday an eight on that scale, we really did have a great day." I finished getting all of the details of Sunday, and we then talked about the rest of the week, and what they would each say happened that they were pleased with. They were noting details and talking about the things during the week that they had enjoyed. They talked about the date they went on to see a movie on Thursday night, spurring another great day of things going well for them, and pointing out – through carefully worded questions on my part – what each would say their partner did to contribute to things going so well during that span of time. Throughout the session both of them relaxed as they gave me these positive details of the week past, and by the end of their descriptions they were sitting closer on the couch and laughing, and easily able to talk about how they would notice that progression continue through the following week – even through some tough conversations they might have, like the one that spurred a fight the day before. They were able to answer these questions as this loving couple who had a better week than they'd had in a long time, and as a result they were able to work through how to move past their disagreement and keep working towards their preferred future.

Richard

Richard is a middle-aged man who had come in with his husband for several sessions previously, and decided to come in for some individual sessions since their relationship got better to work on some personal hopes he had for himself. In this individual session he came in after previously describing his hope as finding some balance in his life. He was incredibly busy and focused, working diligently on a law degree at a local prestigious law school, and he wanted to be sure he was caring for himself, for his family, and for his beloved relationship throughout this very busy and stressful time.

As usual I started the session with "What's been better, since we last spoke?" and Richard immediately said that things were in fact not very good at all. He went on to explain how his schedule had become overwhelming over the last few months, and on top of his crazy and stressful school schedule, his mother, who lived in another state, had just been diagnosed with terminal cancer. Richard tearfully explained the situation to me, and said that for the first time in his life he felt what it must be like to be truly depressed. He said that for about a week or so between our last session and this one, he felt like a heavy jacket had been put on him, and for that week he just wanted to stay in bed and ignore the world around him, a desire that could have put everything he had been working towards at risk if he succumbed. He managed to get up and go to school and take care of his responsibilities, but he said that throughout this time he was so down that he barely even remembered how he got through it. He described fighting tears on his drive into and from school, and feeling sad and anxious throughout every day during that week. As he was talking about this jacket of depression that he wore, he mentioned, as an aside, that one day it seemed to feel a little bit better again, but, he added, he knew that for the foreseeable future this jacket would be something he just had to endure from time to time, and he dreaded the day he woke up wearing it again.

I asked him very carefully about the day he mentioned where he woke up and realized that the jacket was gone, and what he might guess led to that day being better somehow. He immediately said that he thought it was just better that day, not attributing it to anything he did in particular;

it was, he thought, just happenstance. But I sat quietly for just a second longer, allowing him to consider the question some more, and he said, "You know what, I think I do know what happened that might have helped." He went on to explain that the evening before that morning, he did two seemingly normal things but now realized that both of them must have led to his waking up feeling better. The night before he felt better he spoke with his brother about his mother, and they talked for a long while about what was happening with her and how they were going to help her and their father get through this time together. Then he made a decision while talking with him and his husband, to not go to summer school as he was planning, but instead to take the summer off so that he could have time to go and spend time with his parents, to be with his mother, and help his father and brother. He realized then that talking with his family and loved ones was key for him getting through this incredibly tough time, and that taking some things off his plate with the purpose of prioritizing time with them throughout this difficult process with his mother was a very important piece of keeping that jacket of depression at bay – or helping to remove it, should it come back.

Both of these case examples point out how clients often come in and feel as though things are not better, and in that moment they might truly not be. However, with respectful and tenacious questions, a solution-focused therapist can still get the information they are seeking – the seeds that the client has begun to sow towards their preferred future.

Scaling and the next small signs of progress

Once the progress that's been made towards the client's preferred future has been fleshed out, the SF therapist might go back to the scale to see where the client is compared to where they want to be. This scaling looks very much like scaling in the initial session, where you identify current placement and then talk about the next small steps forward. Or the therapist might simply transition into the next small signs of progress through the natural flow of the conversation, without immediately returning to the scale itself.

Here's a transcript where the conversation naturally leads to the next signs of progress without use of the scale:

Session 2: a transcript

I first met with Christina, a young trans-woman, in 2013, after she came in seeking a letter for HRT. She had identified as female for more than a year, and had fully socially transitioned at home, work, and school. She was hoping to begin HRT but wanted to have a couple of therapy sessions to be sure that medical transition was the right path for her. When she came back in two weeks later, here is the conversation we had:

T: So, what's been better since I first saw you a couple of weeks ago?

C: Umm, increased enthusiasm because I have an appointment with a doctor for HRT.

T: OK, so you've got more enthusiasm?

C: Yes, I have, um, my big brother, who I'm not really that close to, came down to take care of some things down here where he has some support, I guess. And, um, he hasn't seen me in three years, and so I took him to lunch and we were talking and he didn't know how to talk with me. So I just opened up the window and said "Just ask anything darling, questions are just curiosity and that's how you gain knowledge." It's about education and that prevents ignorance. And I let him know a lot about who I am now, and what I'm going through. And he's like "It's cool I'm not judging you, it's your life." So yes, he was very accepting and it's just one more supportive person in my life, and I'm so grateful.

T: What do you think it is about you, that engenders such amazing support?

C: I think it's my outlook, one of my outlooks is people are like copy machines, what you put in is what you get out.

T: So what is it that you put in?

C: What makes people comfortable. Kindness, sincerity, and genuineness, that's what attracts people. I think I've perfected it.

T: As evidenced by your family, who has come to bat for you every time you've told them something that may be difficult for some to hear!

C: Absolutely.

T: OK. So enthusiasm has been better. What else has been better since I saw you last time?

C: A better understanding, or a more deep down belief that this is the right path for me because of the fact that it's all coming together so smoothly and so quickly. It's all happening now and without having to wait.

T: How has that been impactful, for this belief to be pounded home for you?

C: I have a lot, well not a lot, but a bit more confidence about whether this is the right path for me or not. But, umm, I've got a lot more cheerful, peaceful feelings inside, that lighthearted peace of mind type thing, that these things are coming together.

T: OK. If I was gonna ask anybody in your life what they've noticed about you, who do you think would be the first person in your life to say that they've noticed that little bit more confidence and peace of mind.

C: Umm...my uncle. I have a gay uncle. [Laughing.]

T: OK.

C: And so I, umm, really look up to him, he knows a lot more than I do, so he really teaches me things and shows me the ropes and whatnot as far as our community, and so I really look up to him and spend a lot of time with him, and so I think he would be the first to point out little changes.

T: What do you think he would point out, if I were to ask him what he's noticed to let him know that though you were already a confident person that confidence has increased in the last couple of weeks. What might he say that he's noticed?

C: Umm...I believe he'd say that I carry myself more like a lady, because over the years I found that gay boys carry themselves a bit differently than actual women. It's fabulous. It's not that I've changed who I am as a person by all means but um yes.

T: So he would say that he's noticed the way you're carrying yourself. Anything else he would say he's noticed? Anything you might guess he would say?

C: I know for a fact that I am different every day. There's not a day that goes by that I'm the same person, so to him I think that's mostly the point that he would make.

T: She's carrying herself more like the woman she is.

C: Yes.

T: OK, can you tell me more about carrying yourself more like "Christina," you said it's different than a gay boy, can you tell me more about that difference, and the impacts of that for you?

C: I use names, I say like what's the difference between "Christopher" and "Christina" and, um, when I really meditate on it, I think of Christopher, and he was always happy and loved to put smiles on other people's faces, and with Christina, I can say that she's a little bit quieter, and wiser, definitely wiser, and yes...they are the same person all in all, it's just who I used to be and who I am now.

T: Yeah...so keep describing Christina to me, quieter, wiser...

C: Umm...Christina is, uh, I couldn't ask for more, if I was to look at myself in a mirror she's a supermodel, she has dreams and goals for herself, and she loves to prioritize and keep on the right track basically. Keep the ones who matter the most first.

T: The ones who matter most?

C: Yeah, my family and friends and of course myself, prioritizing them and keeping those relationships strong.

T: OK. How else have you seen this evolution that you're describing a little bit, besides making a doctor's appointment and carrying yourself differently, that gives you evidence that this evolution is absolutely happening.

C: This session, the sessions that I have here are very helpful, and help me to see this realization because you know other people ask me, when did you decide to become transgender. I recently had this young man who wanted to date me ask me the same question and I answer everyone the same, "I don't see it in any way as a decision, it's mostly a realization and I came to this realization shortly after high school and I started getting into my passion." Because I've always had a passion for female impersonation and drag and the stage, and my stage name, I picked "Christina" and shortly over time it really…I cannot explain…it really began to be a new beginning, like opening old suitcases and finding treasures about myself.

T: Tell me more about what you're finding about yourself, I mean you already started making a list of attributes. What else are you pulling out of that treasure chest?

C: Let me see, umm…I've become more and more of an activist. 'Cause I have a lot of gay and lesbian friends and trans friends…so I love to motivate. I see the LGBT community as rare, and everyone else is 'common'…so friends come to me and seek advice. So I have a friend, who is my gay sister, and she is always trying to walk in my shadow, and I say "look at your shadow honey, there's no difference."

T: Mm hmm. So you've found the helper, the leader, the activist and the motivator?

C: Yes.

T: What else are you pulling out of that chest?

C: Umm…let me see….a deep love for myself, more and more.

T: And how are you noticing the confidence and self-love playing itself out? Like if I were to see you on a day before you opened this treasure chest, and I were to see you today, what differences would I notice that would give me evidence of that confidence and self-love?

C: I would look different, physically.

T: OK so the physical evolution?

C: Yes.

T: You're caring for yourself physically in a different way?

C: Absolutely…I mean I really had characteristics like my father and now I can compare myself to other girls.

T: OK so how would you know, leaving here, if this confidence, and maturity, and self-love were continuing to be a part of you as you take the next steps in your journey towards becoming your true self? What do you imagine would be happening next as these things continue to play a vital role in your life as you move forward?

C: I think that these traits will help me with my transition. My mom told me that she saw a talk show with a transgender female and she learned about how much depression that girl went through, and my mom said she doesn't want that for me. And I told her that if it comes to play, you know, than that is a sacrifice that I'm more than willing to make, because just because I'm going through this chemical change it doesn't take away from this knowledge that I have or this self love that I have for myself. And these traits that I have will help me and my family should the transition become challenging for me or for them.

T: Wow. So you wanted your mom to know that even if you do go through difficult emotional phases with this transition, your strengths will help get you through?

C: Absolutely.

T: And how do you think your mom would notice that being true?

C: I would talk to her, I would be honest with her when I was going through a tough time, or having a difficult day. She would notice that I might feel sad, or upset, or be having a bad day, but I was still living life, going to work and school, and being honest with her about what I was feeling.

T: What difference would that make, to continue living life and being honest about what you're going through when things are hard?

C: I think it would let her know that I was going to be OK, and it would help me feel better, talking to her, and moving forward through my day, rather than staying in bed and hiding.

Feedback and closing in subsequent sessions

Once you've identified what's been better, outlined specifically how the client has achieved that progress, and talked with the client about how they would notice continued forward movement towards their preferred future, you get back to the feedback and closing piece of the session. This piece looks a little different in that the feedback given at this point is much more of a summary of the session that just took place, where the clinician summarizes the progress made and what they've learned the client has done to achieve such progress. Closing the session, however, looks almost identical to the first session wherein the clinician simply asks the client to do more of what works and keep noticing what helps things move forward.

Follow-up with April

When I saw April for the second time, a month after our first visit, she reported that she was feeling more confident than she ever remembered feeling in her life. She noticed that her ability to be confident and happy with herself was at an all-time high, and the effects of that were noticeable throughout every aspect of her life. She was at an eight on her scale. She was confident at her new job; she was taking great care of herself, and continuing to experiment with new ways of moving towards her true self with a lot of success. She even noticed something surprising about herself; she said that for as long as she could remember she had this nervous habit of picking at her fingers and her nails. She said she had small sores and calluses all over her fingers as a result of this lifetime habit she'd created, but in the last month she had inexplicably stopped doing this and her hands were never healthier. She had also completely quit smoking in that month, and started exercising regularly.

She had reached such a high point that she thought she was ready to begin HRT, so I wrote her a letter and she was off to take that step. However, when she began taking hormones to help her body begin to fully transition, she realized that her calm, confidence, and happiness were beginning to dissipate. So at our third session – about three months from the day we'd first met – rather than meeting with April, I met with Adam. In that session Adam asked me to use his legal name and male pronouns. I, of course, obliged him, and he said that he was definitely a little bit confused, but even more happy and confident than he'd ever been.

Adam had made so many changes in his life, mentally and physically before beginning hormones, that he was at his absolute best when he started HRT – which allowed him to realize when he began experiencing anxiety and depression again, that the hormones were having this adverse affect, and he figured out that maybe he wasn't truly a trans-woman but rather a genderqueer male who sometimes expressed himself in very effeminate ways, such as female clothing (which he was confidently wearing in that session), manicured nails, and even facial hair removal, which he was quite pleased with.

Now, I will clarify here that this is not a common occurrence. As a matter of fact Adam is the only client I have had, to date, who began HRT and then suspended it quickly, realizing that he may not be truly transgender. Every other individual I've followed up with has been helped significantly by HRT and transition. But with Adam, his success after our first session led to his happiness and confidence reaching a level he never expected, and as a direct result he knew immediately that HRT was having negative effects on him and was able to stop taking it and go back to feeling happy and confident again.

Adam's case reiterates the incredible importance of leading from behind by allowing the client to remain firmly in the driver's seat of solution-focused conversations, with the freedom to discover what works and what doesn't as it relates to their preferred future, without assumptions about what that will look like.

With things as fluid as gender and sexuality, sometimes clients jump to the wrong extreme conclusions about what is really going on with them, when the reality lies somewhere in the middle. Sometimes people who are bisexual or pansexual believe for a time that they are truly concretely gay or straight, until they fall in love with someone who proves that assumption wrong. The lesson here is to stay right where your client is, never going ahead of them with assumptions about what will get them to their preferred future or what it will look like. Because until they are there, you can just never know.

Conclusion

Similar to every first session starting with some form of a description of hope, every second and subsequent session starts with some form of a description of progress. And similarly to how first sessions then detail the preferred future, the second sessions then detail the progress and how it played a part in things moving forward in a way that was right for that client. From that moment in the session, the first and subsequent sessions look very similar, scaling where things are today, and describing then the next small steps forward. And whether this is session number 2 or session number 200, the tasks of each are the same.

Conclusion

> And what's the definition of a good life? I made some difference. That's it.
> If I could just say that. I've made some difference because I've been here
> in this world. Life is a little bit better and I contributed to that. I think
> that would be a good life.
>
> (Insoo Kim Berg, cited in Yalom and Rubin, 2003)

Working, writing and teaching at this intersection is the most rewarding
aspect of my life. I honestly feel as though this is why I was put on
this earth. I cannot express (though I hope this book has helped) how
incredibly passionate I am about both SFBT and the LGBT community. It
is also an incredibly difficult intersection to write a book about because
I am constantly evolving as a therapist, so what I write today I might be
apt to change tomorrow, and the LGBT community is evolving every day
as well.

Within seven days of the very date that I'm wrapping this book up,
Bruce Jenner (now, Caitlyn) has come out as transgender on national TV
in an interview that is having huge tidal wave-sized impacts both on this
community and on my practice, and the Supreme Court of the United
States is hearing arguments that could impact my ability to finally be
legally married in my home state at the age of 36, which will also have
effects on this community and my practice.

As for my evolution, I've (hopefully) got a long way to go in my career,
and I want to grow and do better every single day. If I look back at this
book in five years, or hell, even one year, and feel 100 percent the same
about therapy then as I do right now, I will be incredibly disappointed
that I haven't evolved as a therapist.

Writing this book has been the most incredibly difficult and
nerve-racking thing I have ever done. I started on this journey a couple
of years ago, and went through one of the most trying years of my life
while creating this piece of work. But in the end I look at the quote above
by the woman who played such an important role in creating the thing
I believe I was born to do, and I realize that although there may be those

who don't agree with what I do or how I do it, my ultimate hope is that there is a faction of people out there who read this book, this piece of work that I put out into the world like my heart on my sleeve, and find something inside it that helps them to do good work with the LGBT community. I know that I will get criticized, and that there will be people who decide that I'm doing it all wrong, or at least some of it, but if there are a few who are genuinely helped by this writing, and the LGBT community benefits in some way from this book becoming a reality, then I will have met my goal.

References

Anthony, R. (1999). *Think Big: A Think Collection*. New York: Berkley Books.

Berg, I.K., and Dolan, Y. (2001). *Tales of Solutions: A Collection of Hope-Inspiring Stories*. New York: WW Norton & Co.

Berg, I.K., and Steiner, T. (2003). *Children's Solution Work*. New York and London: Norton.

Connie, E. (2013). *Solution Building in Couples Therapy*. New York: Springer Publishing Company.

De Jong, P., and Berg, I.K. (2008). *Interviewing for Solutions* (3rd edition). Belmont, CA: Thomson Brooks/Cole.

de Shazer, S., and Fiske, H. (2005). *Tapping into Hope. Brief Therapy Network Annual Conference of the Art of Solution-Focused Brief Therapy*. New York: Hayworth.

de Shazer, S., Dolan, Y.M., Korman, H., Trepper, T.S., McCollum, E.E., and Berg, I.K. (2007). *More than Miracles: The State of the Art of Solution-Focused Brief Therapy*. New York: Haworth Press.

Diamond, L. (2008). *Sexual Fluidity: Understanding Women's Love and Desire*. Cambridge, MA: Harvard University Press.

Duncan, L., Ghul, R., and Mousley, S. (2007). *Creating Positive Futures: Solution Focused Recovery from Mental Distress*. London: BT Press.

George, E., Iveson, C., and Ratner, H., (2010). *Briefer: A Solution Focused Training Manual*. London: BRIEF.

    & Ratner, H., (2011). *Briefer: A Solution Focused Training Manual*. London: BRIEF.

Hoff, C.C., Beougher, S.C., Chakravarty, D., Darbes, L.A., and Neilands, T.B. (2010). Relationship characteristics and motivations behind agreements among gay male couples: Differences by agreement type and couple serostatus. In *AIDS Care*, 22(7), pp. 827–835. doi:10.1080/09540120903443384

Iveson, C., George, E., and Ratner, H. (2012a). *Brief Coaching: A Solution Focused Approach*. London: Routledge.

    & Ratner, H., (2012b). *Solution Focused Working*. London, England: BRIEF.

Kalam, A. (2013). *My Journey: Transforming Dreams into Actions*. New Delhi: Rupa Publications India.

Kim, J.S. (2013). *Solution-Focused Brief Therapy: A Multicultural Approach*. Los Angeles: SAGE Publications, Inc.

Kort, J. (2008). *Gay Affirmative Therapy for the Straight Clinician: The Essential Guide*. New York: WW Norton & Company.

Lipchik, E. (2002). *Beyond Technique in Solution Focused Therapy: Working with Emotions and the Therapeutic Relationship*. New York, NY: Guilford Press.

National Center for Lesbian Rights (2015). #BornPerfect: The Facts About Conversion Therapy. (2015). Retrieved April 25, 2015, from: www.nclrights.org/bornperfect-the-facts-about-conversion-therapy/

Orlick, T. (2008). *In Pursuit of Excellence* (4th edition). Champaign: Human Kinetics.

Schuller, R. (1983). *Tough Times Never Last, But Tough People Do!* Nashville: T. Nelson.

Solomon, S.E., Rothblum, E.D., and Balsam, K.F. (2005). Money, housework, sex, and conflict: Same-sex couples in civil unions, those not in civil unions, and heterosexual married siblings. In *Sex Roles*, 52, pp. 561–75.

Students' Academy (2014). *Words of Wisdom: Abraham Lincoln*. Lulu.com.

Students' Academy (2015). *Words of Wisdom: Robert Louis Stevenson*. Lulu.com.

Taylor, P. (2013). *A Survey of LGBT Americans: Attitudes, Experiences and Values in Changing Times*. Washington, DC: Pew Research Center.

Vos Savant, M. (2014, October 31). Developing Your Strengths. Retrieved May 11, 2015, from: http://parade.com/350733/marilynvossavant/developing-your-strengths-2/

Witkin, S.L. (1999). *Questions* (editorial). *Social Work*.

Yalom, V., and Rubin, B. (2003). Insoo Kim Berg on Brief Solution-Focused Therapy. Retrieved May 11, 2015, from: www.psychotherapy.net/interview/insoo-kim-berg

Zeig, J.K., and Gilligan, S.G. (eds). (2013). *Brief Therapy: Myths, Methods, and Metaphors*. New York: Routledge.

Index

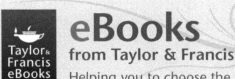

Lightning Source UK Ltd.
Milton Keynes UK
UKHW051159070419
340596UK00012BA/187/P